Book Reviews

"You have to read this book! Probably the best book on health I have ever read. I have no background in nutrition or science but I was so impressed that I shared this book with my immediate family, as it has great advice that will help them have a healthier and happier life. Anyone, no matter if you are vegetarian or a meat eater, can benefit from this invaluable information. Highly recommended for anyone who has even the remotest interest in the world around us and the survival of the human species!!"

Edwin Lugo, Lt. Col., USAF, Ret.
Tampa, Florida

"Despite my skepticism, I found your book inspiring, encouraging, and thought provoking. It leaves me with not only questions about the current research state, but also self-reflections regarding my own eating habits. I believe this is an essential goal of your book: encourage readers to think about health and nutrition regardless of personal beliefs and pre-existing conceptions. Hence, I believe reading your book would benefit a lot of people as an informative holistic approach to health and nutrition and as rising self-awareness of the effect of poor eating habits and modern nutritional deceptions. Your opinions delivered with the right dose of humor and regardless of whether one may agree, question, or disagree, open a much-needed debate on health and nutrition and serve the honorable purpose of raising awareness, which often is the foundation of change. I applaud your efforts and persistence into sharing your knowledge and findings."

Severine C. J. Murdoch, Ph.D., Consule Honoraire de France
Dubois, Wyoming

"I love this book! I really do. Filled with insight, wisdom, humor and practical recommendations that could literally save your life and definitely extend it. Everyone, no matter your background or education level, can get great information from this work. We must all wake up to the realities you present and become conscious of our genetic potential and how to reach it. You lay out our current condition through mind-blowing facts and show the way to healing through the latest nutritional science. Kudos to you and your brilliant work."

Tonja Waring, The Manifesting Mindset
Dallas, Texas

"This book is full of spectacular and break-through medical and nutritional practices that will influence your health both short term and long term in a positive way. As a result of Dr. Arbetter's cogent advice, I have managed to understand how inflammation can be controlled and blood pressure maintained. The ideas are simple but very well researched with the latest in medical and nutritional advances that come from refereed material and Dr. Arbetter's ability to translate this source information to layperson's terms--simple and direct. This book is literally life changing and shall be consulted for myself and others for many years to come."

Dean F. Osgood (Lt Col ret), BS in Engineering, MS in Administration, MS in Program Management, and Level III DAWIA-qualified in Program Management
Springfield, Virginia

"This incredibly well written treatise on health, nutrition, and well-being is not for everyone. For those who will read it (and you may need a medical dictionary or someone who speaks "medical") there is much to glean from it. While I don't necessarily agree with everything here, I respect what is written and its basis in science. I highly recommend the chapter on hydration. Something we all take for granted but should not. Even though I am not (nor will ever be) a true vegetarian, little less a vegan, I can appreciate the points raised. From reading Bob's book I know I will eat better and be more conscious of what I do eat. In conclusion, a totally worthwhile, challenging read. For those who can digest the information, and there is a lot, I believe you will have much to think about and many changes to make."

Randy Shulkin, Pharmacist
Dallas, Texas

Client Testimonies

"I have been suffering with stomach and abdominal issues (intense cramping and bloating) which would sometimes trigger other issues throughout my body since I was 26. These issues were so bad that I consulted multiple doctors to find the source. I spent five years with multiple doctors and have been through multiple operations with no results or explanation to show for it. In 2014, I had the pleasure of meeting Dr. Arbetter through a co-worker of mine and had an enlightened conversation about how the body functions to include the stomach. Within 30 minutes of the conversation, Dr. Arbetter identified what my previous doctors did not by looking at me as a whole and evaluating my overall lifestyle. He explained that the symptoms I was experiencing throughout my body were related to the issues I was having with my stomach. My stomach was the key, he further explained what happens when it is not operating at 100% and how to correct it.

Dr. Arbetter created a custom plan after identifying, without tests, that my diet and long history of taking pain killers slowly deteriorated the ability for my body to process food properly. His plan systematically identified foods that caused my stomach issues while changing my diet to allow my stomach to heal. Within weeks, I noticed a difference. I found foods like wheat, barley and rye greatly contributed to my discomfort and that by taking a balanced mix of vitamins, pre-biotics, probiotics, and enzymes, I could start the healing process. By removing certain foods and altering my diet to include healthier choices I was completely pain free.

After a year, I was able to reintroduce the foods back into my diet with minimal issues.

I still continue to use his advice today and owe him a debt of gratitude for removing this source of pain and discomfort in my life. I highly recommend consulting with Dr. Arbetter for nutritional and advice. His holistic approach to life is refreshing and enlightening."

Rob Wible, Los Angeles

"I spoke with Dr. Arbetter about my growing hip discomfort and the effect it was having on my mobility and enjoyment of various activities, not to mention just walking to and from my car at work. He suggested several things including modifications to my diet to reduce inflammation and several supplements. I put his advice to the test and found a great deal of relief. I especially found the supplement Ceytl Myristoleate (CMO) to be helpful. Approximately a month after starting the recommended protocol of CMO, I experienced significant relief. While being diagnosed (x-ray) by an orthopedist with an arthritic hip, the recommendations Dr. Bob suggested seem to have gotten me back to a level of mobility and pain relief I haven't experienced for over a year. I only wish I had started this routine at the first hint of problems."

Brian, California

"Bob Arbetter knows his stuff. A couple of months ago I was feeling very fatigued and sluggish even though I had been exercising three times a week. In addition, my blood pressure was still high on some days even though I was taking daily medication for it. I mentioned all of this to Bob, and he immediately asked me to describe for him my diet and how much water I consumed daily. He pointed out to me that my diet was high in salt since I ate a lot of snacks and ate substantial amount of processed food. Furthermore, he pointed out that I drank too much diet soda. I decided to follow his advice by reducing my snacking, eliminating completely the diet soft drinks, and reducing the amount of processed foods that I ate. The results of all of this was quick and outstanding. My blood pressure came down to normal and my energy level increased enormously. I guess it is true what they say: "You are what you eat." Thank you, Bob, for reminding me of this and for moving me in the right direction."

Ray, Northern Virginia

"I have been working with Bob Arbetter for about six months. His expertise and knowledge in natural and alternative health is impressive. As my Chiropractor said following a discussion of Bob's recommendations, "Wow, this guy really knows his stuff". In addition to being a very knowledgeable practitioner, he is kind, respectful and compassionate.

I have the highest respect and gratitude for Bob and his determination and wisdom in his field. I recommend Bob Arbetter to anyone fortunate enough to have the opportunity to work with him-you will be so glad you did."

Susan Manning, Austin
LPC, MSW-ACP, LMFT

"Bob is truly excellent as a nutritional healer. Following his advice, in six months, I was able to lower my cholesterol about 60 points. In that time, I progressed from where my doctor was recommending I take statin medications, to where I had very healthy numbers. I also lost about 25 pounds by following Bob's eating recommendations.

Bob worked with me over the phone and mostly by email, as we live in different states. He was always available when I needed him and responded with all kinds of good ideas and inspiration to every issue that I had throughout the process. He is knowledgeable about treatments for all kinds of health issues and aches and pains one might have. He is still following-up with me to maintain my progress and help with a few other issues he is working to help me solve.
Bob really cares about helping people and devotes a lot of time to patients. His wide range of knowledge and education in biology, chemistry and natural health, means that I feel comfortable and trust the things he suggests. When he occasionally has an idea, I do not want to try, he always comes back with alternatives for me. Any questions I have are answered and explained in detail. Bob is incredibly knowledgeable, insightful, and dedicated. I enthusiastically recommend Bob to anyone wanting excellent and expert natural alternative health care.

Gail, Dallas

"I am very appreciative of the coaching you have given me over the years. When we started working together, I was flatly exhausted, in fact completely wiped out after my bike rides. I usually rode about 42 miles and then had to rest or sleep most of the afternoon. Once we started working together, you changed what I ate the night before, what I ate the morning of my rides, the recovery powder I used after my rides and the bars I ate during my rides.

Now, I can ride 50 miles easily, feel no energy drain at all and come home totally refreshed. In fact, last Saturday when I got home, my wife wanted to go on an hour walk. I changed clothes and took off. I feel great now after my rides, in fact, it feels like I haven't done anything at all.

Jay, Dallas

"I decided to lose weight for a lot of reasons. I was limited in the kinds of activities that I could enjoy, the kinds of clothes I could wear, and I felt like the person I am was not adequately reflected through my outward appearance. I ate out so much that several restaurants even had my order memorized. Everything I cooked at home tasted terrible. My medical conditions included sleep apnea, spinal injury from a motor vehicle accident, post-herpetic neuropathy from shingles, severe cystic acne, and endometriosis (a condition that affects fertility). In October 2013, I was 28 years old and 212 pounds, the heaviest I remember being. When I decided to start losing weight, I met with my doctor, bought an elliptical machine for my living room and began counting calories. My original goal was to lose 60 pounds in one year. I thought I was putting a lot of effort into my weight loss, but I didn't see the results I was hoping for. It took me eight months to lose 20 pounds.

I started working with Bob in August 2014. Bob has helped me learn new things about nutrition as well as reaffirm some things that I had known. For example, not all oils are created equal – and this really does matter. Bob helped me re-start my effort, and we created a nutrition and exercise plan that included physical and psychological goals. Bob is very knowledgeable in exercise and nutrition that is focused on minimizing extra fat stores. My goal has always been to slim down without putting on massive amounts of muscle. I am achieving that goal and gaining strength and stamina. I like the way I look, and I feel great. Most importantly, I am armed with knowledge and tools to succeed for a lifetime. Bob has coached me through a major surgery and several re-starts to my nutrition plan.

One of the most important ways that Bob has helped me is in the area of getting back on track. My food addictions to sugar, sweets, meat, as well as my minimally active lifestyle, have at times slowed my progress. When Bob suggests trying something new, I trust him because his advice works. He has helped me brainstorm what I could switch out in place of cake and donuts– it tastes just as good and is also good for me. I am no longer afraid of the so-called "plateau" because I am better equipped to break any plateaus. I have a deeper understanding of the benefits and tradeoffs of different kinds of fasts.

I enjoy talking with Bob about micronutrients in foods. He introduced me to the great benefits of green smoothies. Nowadays, I have a smoothie at breakfast and also one at dinner. A key for me was when he told me that the smoothie really should taste good – this was good news! If it tastes good, I'm more likely to keep doing it. Dieting is not about being hungry and limiting foods. It's about exploring new foods, trying new cooking techniques, finding nutrients that are deficient, and keeping everything delicious. Bob also helped me with food combinations, probiotic selection, cleansing, and acne among many others.

I am now 151 pounds. I met my weight loss goal to lose 60 pounds. I am no longer clinically obese. My acne is cleared. I have a great outlook and maybe a marathon in my future.

Jennifer, Boston

CONNECTING THE DOTS

Reclaiming Your Health, Power,
Clarity and Brilliance

Bob Arbetter, PhD

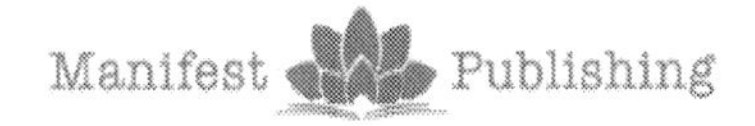

To order copies in quantities, contact Dr. Bob Arbetter at
justbob3@verizon.net

ISBN—978-1-944913-47-2

CONTENTS

INTRODUCTION

It was a typical work day, I put on my suit as normal, kissed my wife, pet the dogs and left for work. I arrived at my office early in the morning and started pulling all my work out of my safes so I could continue with my analysis of the Army intelligence budget.

I was an Air Force full Colonel working in the Pentagon for the Secretary of Defense as his Imagery Intelligence Account Manager; it was my job to balance all activities across the department that had to do with Imagery Intelligence from a financial perspective. On top of that, I was also working with the entire Intelligence Community (all 16 agencies) so that we were coordinated and joined at the hip on putting forth a cohesive intelligence budget to the President and Congress.

Working at that high of a level, they did not want me wearing a uniform. I was one of a handful of rankless agents of the Secretary of Defense; there to do a job and deal with people of all ranks. No one could give us any crap because we were too low or too high in rank. They knew exactly the power of the office we represented.

My kind were not exactly well liked; we were the 60-minutes staff of the department.

They knew if they did not cough up their data, we would still come out with our analysis and recommendations as best we could on insufficient data, and they would not like those results. So, they were best off cooperating. When we showed up, it meant we were going to get into your financial knickers, take a good hard look, and most likely, you would end up with less money to do an already impossible task with the money you had.

But on the other hand, while the right hand taketh, the left hand giveth. So, if you happened to be on the receiving end, I was your best friend. You never knew which way the axe was going to fall until I made my recommendations to the Secretary of Defense, and they submitted their balanced proposal to Congress (after White House adjustments, of course).

I will never forget my boss. He was a wonderful, brilliant PhD in applied mathematics. He had a heart of gold and yet was tough as nails when it came to a fight over money. I would hate to go up against him in an open debate on any subject. That particular morning for no apparent reason, he started yelling for everyone to come into his office. There, he sat glued to the only television. Nobody said a word as we all gathered and witnessed the unbelievable – two planes plowing into the Twin Towers in New York City. Today, was the infamous 9/11.

We were in disbelief along with the entire world.

After watching this terrible tragedy for several minutes, if it seemingly couldn't get any worse, all hell broke loose. The third plane had hit the Pentagon. There was screaming and yelling as people panicked and ran for their lives. Because of our location in the building, we were able to lock up our files before exiting the building, but our roof was on fire and a large mushroom cloud was building over our famous site.

The security guards were yelling at us to get the hell out of there and directing us to safety. At the same time, some ignored the security guards and went the other direction, straight into the disaster. These guards and people running towards the disaster deserve our highest respect; they saved many lives that day. They completely ignored the possibility of personal injury or death to see if they could help others in any way.

Most of the people going towards the disaster were Navy. I asked one of my Navy friends how they had the presence of mind to run towards the disaster, and he told me that is how they are trained on a ship. If the ship goes down, they all go down, so everyone is trained to race towards the emergency and get it under control.

I, on the other hand, along with my office mates, followed directions and left through the nearest exit. When I got out, I looked up and saw a four-engine prop plane flying low over the Pentagon and for an instant, thought that a terrorist had dropped a bomb on us, especially with the huge mushroom cloud reaching high into the sky.

I wanted to borrow a cell phone to call my wife, let her know I was alive, but all the networks were jammed and no one was getting through. I suspected they would be closing off the parking lot and we would all be stranded there for hours; I went to my car and left for home. I was hoping that I could keep my wife from suffering too much over the thought of me dead or alive.

Although she was near panic when I got home, I told her to quickly grab the dogs (we had no kids living with us) and some basics because we were under attack. With one plane still not accounted for, we had to leave the D.C. area until that last plane showed up. We drove and drove to get out of town. It was surreal to see folks out on the golf courses we drove past, completely oblivious to what was going on. Finally, the terrible news came; the last plane tragically hit the ground. We went home.

To write these words, even now many years later, still gives me the willies. Little did I know that morning, my life would change forever; I would face five years of PTSD and emotional recovery.

Connecting the Dots

After many studies, interviews and investigations, it was determined that we knew quite a bit of information that could have led us to the discovery of this evil plot, but that we did not have the ability to connect all the information residing in various arms of the federal and local governments. They called this, Connecting the Dots. Ever since then, the intelligence community has been working to break down those barriers and get better at sharing data.

Being an intelligence insider, I could certainly write a book about how far we have come in the area of sharing data, but that is not my objective for writing this book. I want to apply what I've learned and address a more important topic: human health.

After I retired from the Air Force with a BS in Biology from Texas A&M and a never-ending love of science, I went back to school and got my PhD in the Philosophy of Natural Health. Just as the intelligence field failed to connect the dots to produce and prevent a major disaster, so have we failed to connect the dots to prevent disease and sickness that cause way more suffering and casualties than the events of 9/11 ever did.

It is time we wake up and become conscious of the horrible nutritional landscape we all live in, the impact it is having, and how to take action and make better choices to prevent personal disaster and suffering. Like the Navy, we want to run towards the disaster vs. find the quickest exit.

This is why I wrote this book, to identify the dots, how they connect and to help save humanity from itself by making the best choices under the umbrella of awareness, becoming "conscious" of what it takes for us all to wake up and take action to live our full potential as God meant for us.

It's also why I formed a company called the Conscious Health Club. The goal here is for you to reach your maximum allowed age from your genetic potential, age gracefully without disease and even extend your lifespan with modern antiaging science.

The good news is: information is plentiful now.
The bad news is: information is plentiful now.

And, much of it is conflicting.

It takes a well-educated researcher like me to decipher nutritional studies and pull out the value, especially if they are funded by an institution with their profits based on research outcomes from the study. I believe there is value in every study, no matter who funded it. However, consider the source and proceed accordingly. Your overall judgment may be: they ignored this or that or their population size was not large enough, or they were too generalized to draw any specific conclusions, or they have inbuilt bias or the research was funded by a biased organization or that there were too many confounding issues, or correlation does not equal causation. So be it. You learned something you can apply to the next study you read.

Confused people do nothing. All this information can leave you wondering what to do so you end up doing nothing. I have unscrambled much of this for you and provide easily digestible, useable and practical information for the lifestyle choices you make every single day of your life. You cannot avoid making choices so as long as you are at it, you might as well make the best choices possible. This is not a scientific paper here with appropriate citations. I simply cite where I obtained information from major info sources.

Now, I am going to ask one thing of you. If you find this information valuable, please pass it on, recommend it to someone you know, sick or healthy. Please help me to get the word out and enter the mindset of prevention vs. the mindset of treatment. I am communicating, synthesizing, pulling together parts of the health equation to connect the dots and get you on the path to a healthier life, prevent suffering and extend your health and life spans. Are you with me?

Dr. Bob Arbetter
President and CEO, Conscious Health Club, LLC
Website: www.conscioushealthclub.com
Email: bob@conscioushealthclub.com.

PROLOGUE

I was walking down my corral fence line one day and out of the blue, just fell to the ground for apparently no reason. Laying there in the grass I thought, "That's weird." I got up. Looked around. No holes or rocks or anything else. I just fell. "Very strange," I thought.

Then a few months later, I started losing weight uncontrollably and having serious joint pains. Now, I was starting to get worried. Instead of being a strong, healthy 130 pounds at 5'6", I weighed in at 117 pounds and looked emaciated. The doctors were very concerned but had no clues, especially since I had not changed anything in my diet. I spent months visiting all kinds of doctors but didn't fall under any diagnostic categories; I felt helpless.

Finally, a nurse practitioner told me about a naturopath at their clinic and that he had helped a lot of people. "Maybe he can figure it out," she said.

So, in I go for an appointment and he runs a food sensitivity test on me among other blood tests. "Hmmm," he said on the second visit, as he scratched his chin and looked at the results. I was 52 at the time and up until then was a very active, energetic, strong human being. "I think you have a gluten issue," he concluded.

"Really?" I replied. "I've been eating gluten all my life with no problems. How can that be?"

"Well, you're way over reactive to too many foods, telling me that you have gut permeability issues, which in most cases is caused by gluten. Plus, gluten can cause joint pain as well in some people. It can build over time. Let's try getting off gluten for a couple of months and see how you do."

Two months later, I was back to my normal weight, joint pains were almost gone. I could not believe after months of visiting doctors with apparently nothing wrong with me and yet looking like I left a concentration camp, that a simple thing like removing gluten from my diet could change the course of my life.

With a B.S. in biology and a scientist at heart, I changed all my thinking about health and realized that pharmacology and the medical profession has a lot to learn. That restarted my education into the natural, holistic, and integrative medicine world. Years later, I received my Ph.D in holistic nutrition and now, at almost 65, through this book, I'm sharing with you, the reader, what I've learned.

CHAPTER 1

The Dots

Let's start with the Dots. Fasten your seat belts because I have been collecting health facts from various reliable sources for many years. I've included the ones I believe are most relevant.

Here we go.

- ✓ Two hundred experimental drugs intended to treat Alzheimer's disease have failed in the past 30 years. Without new therapies, the number of Alzheimer's patients worldwide will increase dramatically by 2050. Results of current research suffice for health care professionals to begin making a series of recommendations to patients on diet, exercise and levels of social engagement that may help prevent dementia. (*Scientific American*, April 2017)

- ✓ Studies from different parts of the world indicate that after age 60, most people have at least one chronic disorder, such as heart disease or diabetes, and a recent population-based study in Sweden found that at 80, only around one out of 10 individuals were free of chronic diseases. Most had two or more chronic illnesses. (*Scientific American*, April 2017)

- ✓ In the U.S., around 32 percent of people older than 85 have received an Alzheimer's diagnosis, often combined with other types of dementia, such as that caused by vascular disease. (*Scientific American*, April 2017)

- ✓ Every 66 seconds, another American over the age of 65 is diagnosed with Alzheimer's dementia. 3.7 million Baby Boomers will turn 65 in 2018. This means we're hurtling head-first into a brain health epidemic of catastrophic proportions. But new research has proven that doesn't have to be the case. (*GreenMed Newsletter* 9/8/2018)

- ✓ Today, 100,000 people in the U.S. are in the ICU right now. The mortality of those is 50%. Only 12% will leave to lead a normal life. The cost of this care is $20 billion. (*New England Journal of Medicine* 2014)

- ✓ Chronic inflammation causes reduced stem cell function in the bone marrow. Since the bone marrow produces cells which enhance the immune system, this leads to reduced T-cells and Natural Killer cells. With decreased immune function, disease risk increases. (Dr. Dip Maharaj, Lecture RAADFEST 2016)

- ✓ The level of sugar in the bloodstream at any given time is maintained at about five grams or one teaspoon. (Dr. Sarah Hallberg, 11/12/16 Fat Summit)

- ✓ Alzheimer's is really a protective reaction against three different conditions; Inflammation, lack of nutrition or buildup of toxins. (Dr. Dale Bredesen, 11/12/16 Fat Summit)

- ✓ The ongoing mass extinction of the species and with it the extinction of genes and ecosystems, ranks with pandemics, world war and climate change as among the deadliest threats that humanity has imposed on itself. (Edward O. Wilson, Harvard University)

- ✓ Aluminum toxicity to the nervous system is documented well back to the 20th century. (Celeste McGovern, *TTAC Newsletter* March 2017)

- ✓ Cancer is now universally recognized as a global epidemic. As of 2012, there were 14 million new cancer cases worldwide, including more than 8 million cancer related deaths and more than 32 million people living with cancer. It is estimated that 1.7 million new cases were diagnosed in the U.S. in 2016 and that around 600,000 Americans died of the disease. National expenditures for cancer care in the U.S. were nearly $125 billion in 2010 and likely to reach $156 billion in 2020. (Dr. Suresh Nair, *TTAC Newsletter* April 2017)

- ✓ It is becoming increasingly apparent that our diet, gut microbiota and health are inextricably linked. We must be conscious that, when we make dietary interventions, we affect the growth of trillions of bacteria. (*Nature*, 11/21/16)

- ✓ There are over 50 diseases associated with microbiota or gut disbiosis. (Michael Ash)

- ✓ Brain cells can grow throughout your life as a result of stress reduction, toxin elimination, low chronic inflammation and diet control. Mother's stress level during pregnancy influences the size of the neocortex in her baby. Factors that influence Neurogenesis (nerve creation): Elimination of bad fats, increased good fats, aerobic exercise, meditation, high levels of

DHA, bioflavonoids like hesperidin, ECGC, quercetin, apigenin, leuteolin, gensing. (Bryant Courtwright, interview with Dave Aspry #287)

- ✓ The National Institute of Health (NIH) says 24 million people in the U.S. have autoimmune disease and we know only one out three have been diagnosed, so 72 million have the disease. Atherosclerosis initiation is an autoimmune reaction to an injured vessel lining. Autoimmune disease is expected to double in 20 years. The cause: exposure to compounds that are integrated into our cells that invite attack from our immune system (gluten, lectins, drugs, toxins, bad oils, etc.) (Dr. Thomas O'Brian, Interview with Sayer Ji 11/11/16)

- ✓ The NIH is now saying there is link between cell phone radiation and cancer. (*UK's Mirror*, 11/7/18)

- ✓ In *World Psychiatry Journal*, Swedish and Finish researchers found that the risk of committing a homicide increases by 31% in patients taking an anti-depressant drug, 45% with anti-anxiety drugs, 206% with anti-inflammatory drugs and 223% with opioid pain killers.

- ✓ Psychiatric drugs are responsible for the deaths of more than a million people aged 65 and older each year in the western world. (*British Medical Journal* 5/12/15)

- ✓ The highest dairy consuming countries in the world are: Sweden, Finland, England, U.S. The highest rates of osteoporosis are in the same countries. Calcium absorption rates are higher in green leafy vegetables than in dairy. (John and Ocean Robbins Food Summit)

- ✓ The Relaxation Response is seen from over 2,209 genes in gene expression of meditators. These genes influence immune responses, inflammation, premature aging including thinning of brain cortex and conditions related to oxidative stress. (Dr. Herbert Benson)

- ✓ Based on estimates, in 2013, the 3rd leading cause of death in the U.S. was medical error. First was heart disease, 2nd was cancer, 4th was COPD, 5th was suicide, 6th was firearms and 7th was motor vehicles. (*British Medical Journal*)

- ✓ Federal recommendations for adult women are at least 1-1/2 cups of fruit and 2-1/2 cups of vegetables each day. Men need at least 2 cups of fruit and 3-1/2 cups of vegetables each day. In a recent Morbidity and Mortality Weekly Report (MMWR) article, Center for Disease Control (CDC) researchers found that only, 9% of adults met the intake recommendations for vegetables and 12% of adults met the recommendations for fruit. (CDC as of 8/6/2018).

- ✓ The brain, which is only 5% of our body weight, consumes 25% of our calories. (Dr. David Perlmutter)

- ✓ There are 800 incidents of DNA damage in our bodies per hour. Out of nine foods tested, six conferred DNA protection: raw lemons, persimmon, strawberry, apple, broccoli and celery. (Dr. Gregor, 5/16/16)

- ✓ It is estimated that after age 40, there is approximately a 20 to 30% decrease in body enzyme production. When uncooked food is consumed, fewer digestive enzymes are required, preserving them to assist in vital cellular metabolic functions.

Cooking foods for long periods of time above 118 degrees destroys enzymes and leads to today's enzyme-less diet. (*Life Extension*)

- ✓ Not a single diet of the big 4-5 have even the minimum amount of the RDA recommended nutritional levels. (Dr. Calton)

- ✓ It is estimated that our hunter/gatherer ancestors got more than 100g per day of fiber. The National Center for Health statistics estimates U.S. averages only 14-15g per day. A study of 43,757 male health professionals revealed that the highest fiber intake (29g/day) were 55% less likely to develop cardio vascular disease. In a study of 68,782 female nurses, 22.9g fiber showed 66% less likely for cardio vascular disease. (Dr. Floyd H. Chilton, *Inflammation Nation*)

- ✓ Telomere length and telomerase activity are factors associated with aging and a number of chronic diseases including hypertension, cardio vascular disease, diabetes Type 2, depression, osteoporosis and obesity. Telomere length can be influenced by diet and lifestyle factors, exercise, fiber intake, vitamins and mineral intake. (Dr. Jeff Bland)

- ✓ We were a hunter/gatherer society for 100,000 generations, an agricultural society for 500 generations and a highly processed food society for two generations. (Dr. Floyd H. Chilton, *Inflammation Nation*)

- ✓ Insulin levels influence the production of inflammatory messengers, which in turn regulate insulin levels. (Dr. Floyd H. Chilton, *Inflammation Nation*)

- ✓ Human clinical trials of 70 trials of 1,000 patients each have shown that 100mg of Curcumin or half a teaspoon of Turmeric is enough to down regulate all known cancers. FDA says it is generally regarded as safe with no known toxic dose. (Dr. Affarwal)

- ✓ The oral microbiome is linked to everything from Alzheimer's to colon cancer. Three studies in 2016 show oral disease is linked to pre-term birth, erectile disfunction, and intercerebral hemorrhage. (Gerry Curatola, DDS)

- ✓ One hundred years ago, the main killer was infectious diseases. Now, it is chronic conditions: heart disease, cancer, stroke and COPD. (Professor Sutterfield)

- ✓ Women with breast cancer who have the highest lignin (like from flax seed) consumption (1/3 mg/day), had a 71% reduction in mortality from breast cancer. (Dr. Fuhrman)

- ✓ Only 2% of our 22,000 genes code for proteins, the rest non-coding DNA is more than any other life form. It is where the regulation of our complexity resides. This "Dark Matter" is inherited and takes its messages from the environment, diet and lifestyle of the person. (2007 Encode Project from NIH/Dr. Jeff Bland)

- ✓ There are two reasons for animal antibiotics in our beef. One is they are raised in terrible conditions and get infections if not for antibiotics. The second is to fatten them up quickly. The CDC warns about drug resistant strains of pathogens killing thousands today. Obesity is on the rise, is this from consuming antibiotics from our meat sources? (Van Hari)

- ✓ The prevalence of obesity was 39.8% and affected about 93.3 million of U.S. adults in 2015-2016. Obesity-related conditions include heart disease, stroke, Type 2 diabetes and certain types of cancer, some of the leading causes of preventable death. The estimated annual medical cost of obesity in the U.S. was $147 billion in 2008 U.S. dollars; the medical cost for people who have obesity was $1,429 higher than those of normal weight. The prevalence of obesity was 35.7% among young adults age 20–39 years, 42.8% among middle-aged adults age 40-59 years, and 41.0% among older adults age 60 and over. The prevalence of obesity was 18.5% and affected about 13.7 million children and adolescents. (CDC Facts, as of 8/6/18)

- ✓ From 1969-2020, the numbers of deaths due to heart disease have declined, even with a growing U.S. population whereas the numbers of deaths due to cancer have almost doubled, even with a slight decline in the number of deaths per person. Projections indicate that cancer will soon become the leading cause of death in the United States. (*Heart Disease and Cancer Deaths, Preventing Chronic Disease*, 11/17/16)

- ✓ A study of one million students in New York showed that students who ate lunches that did not include artificial flavors, preservatives, and dyes did 14% better on IQ tests than students who ate lunches with these additives. (Dr Mercola.com as of 8/8/18)

- ✓ Other articles detail the drugs used in concentrated animal farming operation (CAFO), and the risks this drug-based farming poses to human health. One side effect is the creation of antibiotic-resistant superbugs, which I've addressed on numerous occasions.

Martha Rosenberg also recently highlighted a USDA Inspector General Report, which revealed that beef sold to the public have been found to be contaminated with a staggering 211 different drug residues, as well as heavy metals. (Dr Mercola.com as of 8/8/18)

✓ Depression is a widespread global problem, with over 300 million people dealing with this severe mood disorder today. Even in developed, industrialized countries, depression is rampant. In fact, in the United States, between 2013 and 2016, 8.1% of Americans who were 20 years old and older suffered from depression in a given two-week period. (Mercola.com as of 8/9/18)

✓ In 2017, an estimated 30.3 million people have diabetes in the U.S. (*National Diabetes Statistics Report* 2017

✓ Sixty to 70 million people affected by all digestive diseases with the following specific diseases (National Institute of Health as of 8/9/18):

- Chronic constipation – 63 million (2000)
- Gallstones – 20 million (2004)
- Acid Reflux – 20% of the U.S. population weekly
- Digestive Infections – nonfood borne: 135 million (1998)
- Digestive Infections – food borne: 76 million (1998)
- Hemorrhoids – 75% of people older than 45 (2006)
- Inflammatory Bowel Disease – 1.9 million (2009)
- Crohn's Disease – 359,000 (1998)
- Ulcerative Colitis – 619,000 (1998)
- Irritable Bowel Syndrome – 15.3 million (1998)

- Liver Disease – 3 million (2011)
- Pancreatitis – 1.1 million (1998)
- Peptic Ulcer – 15.5 million (2011)
- Hepatitis B – 800,000 to 1.4 million (2007)
- Hepatitis C – 2.7 to 3.9 million (2007)

✓ Doctors who received the most lavish gifts from pharmaceutical companies prescribed the most expensive medications. Practitioners who received gifts from Big Pharma wrote more than twice the number of prescriptions than those who didn't. (Study in *PLOS One*)

✓ Big Pharma spends almost $250 million a year lobbying Congress to get their way. To put this into perspective, the gun rights lobby spends just $10 million a year. (Chris Kresser 11/28/17)

✓ For the first time in two centuries, the current generation of children in America may have shorter life expectancies than their parents. The prevalence and severity of obesity is so great, especially in children, that the associated diseases and complications – Type 2 diabetes, heart disease, kidney failure, cancer – are likely to strike people at younger and younger ages. (*New England Journal of Medicine* March 2005)

✓ Sperm concentration has fallen by 52% among most Western countries between 1973 and 2011. By 2011, the count had fallen to 47.1 million. The plummet is alarming because sperm concentrations below 40 million per milliliter are considered below normal and can impair fertility. And, the decline has grown steeper in recent years, which means that the crisis is deepening. Sperm count is the canary in the coal mine, says Levine. "There is something very wrong in the environment." (*Newsweek* 9/2/18)

- ✓ Increasing evidence is accumulating for a steady rise in the frequency of autoimmune diseases (AD), in the last decades. In fact, the rise in ADs parallels the surge in allergic and cancer conditions while infections are less frequent in the Western societies, creating the basis for the hygiene hypothesis. Multiple sclerosis (MS), type 1 diabetes (IDDM), inflammatory bowel diseases (mainly Crohn's disease) (IBD), systemic lupus erythematosus (SLE), primary biliary cirrhosis, myasthenia gravis (MS), autoimmune thyroiditis (AT), hepatitis and rheumatic diseases (RA), bullous pemphigoid, and celiac disease (CD) are several examples. Their relationship to socioeconomic status, their rapid increase in developed countries and observations in selected migrant populations, indicate some form of environmental impact, rather than long-term genetic influences which are driving these recent evolutionary processes. Among many others, three major environmental factors, strongly related to socioeconomical status are suspected to drive these phenomena: infections, ecology and nutrition. (*International Journal of Celiac Disease* Vol. 3, No. 4, 2015, pp 151-155. doi: 10.12691/ijcd-3-4-8)

- ✓ Antibiotic resistance is one of the biggest threats to global health, food security, and development today. Antibiotic resistance can affect anyone, of any age, in any country. Antibiotic resistance occurs naturally, but misuse of antibiotics in humans and animals is accelerating the process. A growing number of infections – such as pneumonia, tuberculosis, gonorrhea, and salmonellosis – are becoming harder to treat as the antibiotics used to treat them become less effective. Antibiotic resistance leads to longer hospital stays, higher medical costs and increased mortality. (World Health Organization 2/5/18)

✓ The prevalence of diabetes has been steadily increasing for the past three decades, mirroring an increase in the prevalence of obesity and overweight people. In particular, the prevalence of diabetes is growing most rapidly in low- and middle-income countries. Diabetes is one of the leading causes of death in the world (World Health Organization):

- In 2012 diabetes was the direct cause of 1.5 million deaths. An additional 2.2 million deaths were caused in the same year by higher-than-optimal levels of blood glucose, through an increased risk of cardiovascular and other diseases. Even when blood glucose levels are not high enough to warrant a diagnosis of diabetes damage can occur to the body. The risk of cardiovascular disease rises as blood glucose levels rise.

- There are 2 major forms of diabetes: Type 1 diabetes is characterized by a lack of insulin production and Type 2 diabetes results from the body's ineffective use of insulin. While Type 2 diabetes is potentially preventable, the causes and risk factors for type 1 diabetes remain unknown, and prevention strategies have not yet been successful.

- A third type of diabetes is gestational diabetes: Gestational diabetes is characterized by hyperglycemia, or raised blood sugar, with values above normal but below those diagnostics of diabetes, during pregnancy. Women with gestational diabetes are at an increased risk of complications during pregnancy and delivery. They and their children are also at increased risk of Type 2 diabetes in the future.

- Type 2 diabetes is much more common than type 1 diabetes: Type 2 accounts for the majority of cases of diabetes worldwide. Higher waist circumference and higher body mass index (BMI) are associated with increased risk of Type 2 diabetes, though the relationship may vary in different populations.

- Reports of Type 2 diabetes in children – previously rare – have increased worldwide. People with diabetes can live long and healthy lives when their diabetes is detected and well-managed: A series of cost-effective interventions can help people diagnosed with diabetes manage their condition. These interventions include: blood glucose control through a combination of diet, physical activity and, if necessary, medication; control of blood pressure and lipids to reduce cardiovascular risk and other complications; and regular screening for damage to the eyes, kidneys and feet, to facilitate early treatment.

- Early diagnosis and intervention are the starting points for living well with diabetes: The longer a person lives with undiagnosed and untreated diabetes, the worse their health outcomes are likely to be. Basic technologies such as blood glucose measurement should be readily available in primary health-care settings. Access to essential medicines (including life-saving insulin) and technologies is limited in low- and middle-income countries. Diabetes of all types can lead to complications in many parts of the body and increase the overall risk of dying prematurely. Possible complications include heart attack, stroke, kidney failure, leg amputation (because of infected, non-healing foot ulcers), vision loss and nerve damage.

- Thirty minutes of moderate-intensity physical activity on most days and a healthy diet can drastically reduce the risk of developing Type 2 diabetes.

✓ We carry at least 700 chemicals in our body that were not part of the human body chemistry before the 20th century. Most of these chemicals have not been well studied, and we don't know much about how they affect us. Tests on how synthetic chemicals affect our health are too simplistic and do not represent what is going on in the real world. One single chemical may have no effect on its own. Yet, it may have damaging effects when combined with other chemicals in a so-called 'cocktail'. Even the most complex tests on chemicals done today include no more than a few other chemicals at the same time. In a way, we are all part of a huge uncontrolled "cocktail experiment" involving hundreds of chemicals. (World Counts Website 10/10/18)

✓ As per U.S. Environmental Protection Agency (EPA) estimates, every year in the U.S, 1.2 trillion gallons of sewage from household, industry and restaurants is dumped in to U.S. water annually. Important water contaminants which are manmade include heavy metals, nutrients, microbial pathogens, sediments, organic matter etc. (*Conserve Energy Future*)

- ✓ In 2016, a Harvard study found Perfluoroalkyl substances (PFAS), very harmful manmade chemical substances, in water from 33 of the 50 states and determined that over six million United States residents were affected by these contaminated water supplies. The Ohio River is seriously contaminated because of chemical dumping from the Dupont industry starting in the 1950s.

- ✓ According to the EPA, 44% of assessed stream miles, 64% of lakes and 30% of bay and estuarine areas are not clean enough for fishing and swimming. The EPA also states that the United States' most common contaminants are bacteria, mercury, phosphorus and nitrogen. These come from the most common sources of contaminates, that include agricultural runoff, air deposition, water diversions and channelization of streams.

- ✓ A recent study published in JAMA® estimated that the rate of ADHD in U.S. children is now one in 10. And, the numbers just keep going up. The prevalence of ADHD 20 years ago, in 1998, was nearly half what it is today – 6%. Such a rapid increase means that the cause cannot be genetic. Our genes don't change that fast. It must be environmental. (Chris Kresser 10/26/18)

- ✓ A prominent University of California immunologist, Alan Levin, estimates that one out of three Americans is adversely affected by candida.

- ✓ "Humanity's survival depends on the planet's resources: fish, water, wood, minerals, and arable land. But the replenishment of these goods depends on the world's natural capital: forests, grasslands, topsoil, lakes, rivers, and oceans. Increases in agricultural productivity and the expansion of critical infrastructure have improved the lives of billions of people but have left this natural capital dangerously depleted. As the overall demand for goods and services has continued to grow, human consumption of natural resources has become unsustainable. In 2010, the nonprofit organization the Global Footprint Network calculated that humanity now requires roughly 1.5 earths to sustain its current level of consumption each year. Put another way, humanity now uses up a year's supply of earth's natural resources by mid-August." (Foreign Affairs, March/April 2014)

CHAPTER 2

Connecting the Dots Takeaways

So, what can we learn from the Dots and many more? Here are my strategic takeaways:

- ✓ We live in an increasingly toxic world and can no longer go about our lives, oblivious to these dangers and expect to lead healthy long lives, unless we are blessed with extremely good genetics.
- ✓ Nutritional science is better than it has ever been, although sometimes conflicting. Education is necessary and abundantly available to help us understand these dangers and help us live creative and productive lives.
- ✓ It is not enough to educate ourselves. We must take action! Our bodies are starving from nutritional deficiencies, not calories. We must make "conscious" efforts to bring in the nutrition our bodies need to thrive while avoiding toxins as much as possible and/or constantly eliminating them from our body.

- ✓ Mental health and physical health are related and taking care of only one will not result in success.
- ✓ Gut health and our gut bacteria are one of the great keys to overall health.
- ✓ We are approaching a time (or are already here) of the have and have nots, just like the huge bipolar economic disparity where you lose the great middle class, and the economic and nutritional have nots are related. In nutrition, we will see an increasing number of centenarians, those folks who connect the dots, take action to change their lifestyles and have the resources to keep up with the latest anti-aging science. On the other side will be the majority of folks who either do not connect the dots or take no action to change their nutritional/lifestyle choices or do not have the resources to eat healthy. Don't let the increasing numbers of long-lived people fool us into thinking society as a whole is getting the message.

Unless we turn this around, the human race is in danger, especially with overuse of antibiotics and falling fertility rates.

DISCLAIMER

I am not a medical doctor, so I cannot provide medical advice, diagnose, treat or cure any disease for it would be illegal for me to do so. The information in this book has not been evaluated by the food and drug administration or any other medical body. Information is shared for educational purposes only. You must consult with your doctor before acting on any content in this book, especially if you are pregnant, nursing, taking medication or have a medical condition. Nothing in this book is to be taken as medical advice and those things you choose to follow are at your own risk.

CHAPTER 3

The Laws of Life

So, what do we do to take action? Before we dive in to each of the many aspects of health, such as hydration, fats, the auto-immunity, energy metabolism, inflammation, epigenetics, ketosis, gut health, the gut-brain connection and others, let's get out of the weeds and stay in the clouds for some high-level health philosophy and basic rules for healthy living. Here are some laws of life (I give credit to the great Herbert Shelton for many of these). I am sure there are more. I wish some of our brightest minds in the medical and health world would think about this and publish their health philosophy, their overall strategic guidelines for the human body and mind and what it takes to thrive in today's world. That would make an interesting chapter. Please submit your ideas to me through my website at conscioushealthclub.com.

1. **Life's Great Law**: Every living cell of the organized body is endowed with an instinct of self-preservation, sustained by an inherent force in the organism called vital force or life force. The success of each living organism is directly proportioned to the amount of its life force and inversely proportional to the degree of its activity.

2. **Law of Order**: The living organism is completely self-constructing, serf-maintaining, self-directing, self-repairing, self-defending and self-healing.

3. **The Law of Power**: The power employed and expended in any vital or medicinal action is vital power, that is, power from within and not from without.

4. **The Law of Distribution**: The power of the body whether that power is great or little, is distributed in a manner proportionate to the importance and needs of the various organs and tissues of the body.

5. **The Law of Conservation**: Whenever nutritive abstinence is affected, the living organism's reserves are conserved and economized: living structures are autolyzed in the inverse order of their usefulness, while toxic substances are being eliminated.

6. **The Law of Limitation**: Whenever and wherever the expenditure of vital power has advanced so far that a fatal exhaustion is imminent, a check is put upon the unnecessary expenditure of power; and the organism rebels against the further use of even an accustomed stimulant.

7. **The Law of Special Economy**: The vital organism, under favorable conditions, stores up all excess of vital force above the current expenditures as a reserve fund to be employed in time of special need.

8. **The Law of Vital Accommodation**: The organism will respond to external stimuli in a manner of self-

preservation, which adapts or accommodates itself to whatever influence it cannot destroy or control.

9. **The Law of Stimulation and Dual Effect**: Whenever a toxic or irritation agent is brought to bear upon the organism, the body puts forth vital resistance, which manifests itself in an action at once accelerated but also impaired. This resistance diminishes the bodily power precisely to the degree to which it accelerates action, diminishing vital power.

10. **The Law of Repose**: Whenever action in the body has expended the substance and available energy of the body, rest is induced in order to replenish the body's substance and energy.

11. **The Law of Selective Elimination**: All injurious substances which gain admittance by any means into the living organism are counteracted, neutralized, and expelled as fully as the bodily Nerve Energy supplies allow by such means and through such channels as will produce the least amount of harm to the living structure.

12. **The Law of Utilization**: The normal elements and materials of life are all that the living organism is ever capable of constructively utilizing, whether well or sick.

13. **The Law of Quality Selection**: When the quality of nutriment being received by the living organism is higher than that of the present living tissue, the organism will discard the lower-grade cells to make room for appropriating the superior materials into new and healthy tissue.

14. **The Law of the Minimum**: The development of the living organism is regulated by the supply of that element or factor which is least abundantly provided or utilized. The element or factor in shortest supply determines the amount of development.

15. **The Law of Development**: The development of all or any parts of the living organism is measured in direct proportion to the amount of vital forces and nutritive materials which are directed to it and brought to bear upon it.

16. **(Mine) The Law of Homeostasis or Balance**: When controlling systems or living materials are out of balance, the body will always strive to return to a state of balance, repair and health in all its systems, even if it means causing ultimately the death of the organism in its effort to restore balance.

17. **(Mine) The Law of Equal Resilience, Protection and Recovery**: To protect the body, vital functionality is maintained, such that, chronic unnatural toxin exposure and nutritional deficiency can build for years and not impede daily function until a tipping point is reached. Therefore, full and true recovery with re-establishing prior resilience can take equal time periods.

A lot can be said about each of these and how to obey these laws and optimize them in our daily lifestyle choices. But to save time, I will simply refer back to them as I proceed on through the chapters in this book. But first, I offer a break for those who might enjoy reading some of my deeper thoughts on life and health (Hey, this is my book. I can do this.). If not interested, skip this section and move on to more substantive chapters.

THOUGHT BREAK #1: THE BREATH OF LIFE

Sometimes, I imagine as part of a relaxation exercise (stress reduction is important to your health!!), that when I breathe in slowly, I pull in all the good and energetic powers around the earth. I inhale through my feet and legs and pull the air and power of the earth through my whole body up into my lungs. Once my lungs are as full as they will go, then I exhale, keeping all the good air and energy, and releasing all the toxins in my body and soul, cleansing my body of all the bad stuff.

Well, one time I extended that vision to a broader amount of stuff I inhale. This time, I thought of the energy that created all matter. The absolute which never changes. The original ether from which we all come from that has no beginning and no end. Maybe, I reasoned, if I could get some of that into my system, perhaps I would slow down my own world, keep my body from changing so fast as I march through time. Time, I know is an invention of the relative, and time passage can be fast or slow, depending on my own relative speed. So perhaps, if I absorbed the absolute where there is no time, my body would learn that lesson and keep on truckin' having removed time as an element in my existence and therefore delay aging.

And then, I had the thought that as I breathe in, I am pulling in the universe, and perhaps I am also causing ever so slightly a pull on the fabric of space/time. The breath of one person could not have much effect, but just maybe, ever so slightly, a very small tug occurs as I inhale, I envision, and all the planets, solar systems and galaxies bend my way and are pulled together towards me. Then as I transition to an exhale, they wait to see what happens next, until I finally release my mighty breath and the universe returns to its normal position.

What a fantasy. But a fun one. And then it hit me like a ton of bricks. What if I am the creator of the universe? A breath from me would be pretty powerful. What if the currently expanding universe could be viewed as the creator breathing out, spreading his creative energy from a central point (the big bang several billion years ago), and we are still in the exhale mode with the universe still expanding. Then at some point, as energy finally dissipates, the great inhale begins, and all the universe reverses direction and galaxies start pulling back to the center.

Once all matter is about the size of pin head (like the big bang started), then that massive amount of matter is converted back to only energy, completing the inhale. Then God exhales again, the big bang occurs again and here we go! The universe could be filling a big energy balloon and God could have his mouth on the nipple! And her breath of life, what keeps her engaged and challenged and interested and creative, is the creation of the material universe, a conversion of energy to matter, so that a different form of life begins anew, creating space and time, allowing a relative existence.

Just as we would be essentially dead without breathing, perhaps God needs the universal expansion and contraction just as much, to allow her to create the material world and thereby feed her soul and satisfy her undying need to create, and if that is one of the principal needs of life in the absolute, and our soul is of the absolute, then it should be one of our primary needs as well, and through our breath, gives us the ability to sustain life in the world of the relative so that we can create as well, thereby an extension of God's own creative needs. If that were true and God could observe us, then he could live through us and thereby exponentially expand his own ability to create. Ahhhhhhh, finally, she feels my soul is satisfied.

This was not the first time I had or have read that thought, but this time it came to me as a logical extension of my own breathing. Were we not created in God's image? Perhaps we have similar powers on a smaller scale. I can only believe that had we been educated from birth about how powerful and wonderful we are, God only knows what we would be capable of (I am sure this is literally true). Our beliefs, it seems to me, must create boundaries to our capabilities. The problem is to believe something different, after a lifetime of incorrect teaching and observation of limited thinking, believing something you suspect to be true, but have not been taught it or observed it in others or in our current reality. How does one break away from a lifetime of well-intentioned teaching and begin to create anew? I don't know how to do that, but somehow, I think it holds the key to our soul's and civilization's evolution, salvation and awakening.

OK, so that was pretty deep. Let's get back to the here and now.

CHAPTER 4

The Secrets of Hydration

We know so much more about water now than we have before. For example, did you know that we make our own water? In our energy factories (mitochondria), we take the hydrogen off sugars and fats, combine it with the oxygen coming in from the air we breathe, and produce our own water! This turns out to be a critical function of our energy production process. Why? Because it reduces the amount of deuterium we are exposed to. Deuterium is heavy hydrogen (hydrogen with a neutron in the nucleus of the atom) and our bodies cannot deal very well with this extra massive hydrogen. So, it uses our energy factory to not only produce ATP but also to filter out heavy water. That is how animals in the desert survive. They are very good at making their own water.

Interestingly enough, the lowest levels of deuterium come from fat rather than sugars and proteins. And the best fats to get into your mitochondria for energy production are the shorter chain fats because they are short enough to move through the double walled mitochondria membrane. So, if you want to help your body by limiting your deuterium intake, consume Medium Chain Tryglycerides (MCTs) that come from coconut oil.

Consider drinking only filtered water, especially if it comes from city water due to the contaminants contained in public water supplies these days. I recommend the new AquaTruWater system. Check it out online. Take it one step further and drink that water out of steel /glass/ceramic containers rather than plastics to avoid leaching of toxins from those plastics which can disrupt hormone systems in the body over time.

Here is some other scientific research going on right now with regard to the structure and memory of water. There is very good evidence that water has different structures and therefore memory. Apparently, the best structure for your body and cells is obtained after water passes through a vortex, like swirling pools and eddies you see in a flowing river.

You can buy vortex devices that attach in your water line and structure your drinking water. I have one underneath my sink and just love it. It also is very good for your plants if you are a home gardener. They make the vortex devices for your garden hose as well. I chose the one that is sold by DocofDetox.com.

Another earth-shattering fact of water structure besides the clean and filtered water you drink, is your body makes ordered water called EZ water or Exclusion Zone water. This water is critical to your health in that it helps repair proteins. You have over 100,000 proteins in your body and for various reasons, they can become unfolded and dysfunctional over time (proteins require proper physical folding and shape in order to do their job). That means you lose hormone, digestive, muscle mass, DNA repair and a million other functions over time as they all involve proteins.

As it turns out, your body produces Free Radicals, some of which are damaging but others that send out a frequency that structures the water around it. This ordered water is required to supply the environment within to repair and refold damaged proteins. There are products on the market which can create (EZ) the water for you to help you stay on top of protein repair, like from Eng3, but they are very expensive.

Some health practitioners have these devices in their clinics where you can go in for treatment. But there are many other benefits of water you may not be aware of so:

1. **Water Prevents Dry Mouth:** Water keeps your throat and lips moist and prevents your mouth from feeling dry. Dry mouth can cause bad breath and/or an unpleasant taste. It can even promote cavities.

2. **Water Promotes Cardiovascular Health:** Dehydration lowers your blood volume, so your heart must work harder to pump the reduced amount of blood and get enough oxygen to your cells, which makes everyday activities like walking upstairs – as well as exercise – more difficult.

3. **Water Keeps Your Body Cool:** Your body releases heat by expanding blood vessels close to the skin's surface (this is why your face gets red during exercise), resulting in more blood flow and more heat dissipated into the air, drain you of your energy, eating all of the sugar in your blood and leaving you with not enough to power your cells. When you're dehydrated, however, it takes a higher environmental temperature to trigger blood vessels to widen, so you stay hotter.

4. **Water Helps Muscles and Joints Work Better:** When you're well hydrated, the water inside and outside the cells of contracting muscles provides adequate nutrients and removes waste efficiently so you perform better. Water is also important for lubricating joints. Contrary to popular belief, muscle cramps do not appear to be related

to dehydration, but, instead, to muscle fatigue, according to Sam Cheuvront, Ph.D., an exercise physiologist.

5. **Water Keeps Skin Supple:** When a person is severely dehydrated, skin is less elastic. This is different than dry skin, which is usually the result of soap, hot water and exposure to dry air. And, no, unfortunately, drinking lots of water won't prevent wrinkles.

6. **Water Cleanses Toxins from Your Body:** Your kidneys need water to filter waste from the blood and excrete it in urine. Keeping hydrated may also help prevent urinary tract infections and kidney stones. If you are severely dehydrated, your kidneys may stop working, causing toxins to build up in your body.

7. **Water Reduces Constipation and Helps Toxin Elimination through the Gut**. Your elimination should be effortless, not too loose and not too solid, at least once a day, hopefully twice. Water will hydrate the movements and ease the passage through the entire intestinal tract. And once that operates normally, you are eliminating toxins from the system much more readily as you were designed to do.

You might ask, how do I know I am getting enough water? The answer is, drum roll please…everyone is different. One gauge is how you feel, but that is not reliable. I never knew I was dehydrated all the time until I started drinking large amounts of water. Once my body got used to it, much of my pain left my body, then it started sending me the right signals when I was low on water, saying it was dying for water. But, things like back pain, constipation, joint pain, and heavy heart beats (water dilutes and thins the blood) you will definitely feel or notice so once you start drinking more water, then slack off. Check these symptoms out and see if they get better with more water.

I recommend starting to drink at least one 6-ounce glass of water every hour. (If you have kidney disease, check with your doctor before consuming large water volumes.) You should have to get up about once an hour and hit the restroom. It is not good to sit for more than an hour anyway. Watch your urine color, it should tend towards clear. Keep track of your movements and get them to at least once a day.

If you still cannot do this, then there are other things you can do to get you to be more regular. More on that in future chapters. See how your energy levels are; your aches and pains should be reduced. Everything should work better, and you should feel better. Sometimes, when you are getting hunger signals, they are really thirst signals. Drink a glass of water to satisfy your hunger and see how that feels. If you are trying to lose weight, there are many facets to that. (I have a whole chapter simply on getting to and maintaining your ideal weight.) But certainly, drinking more water and ingesting fewer calories can help. Plus, once you get to be more regular, it will help with weight loss, because one reason you retain fat is to store toxins. The more you move toxins out of the body, the more it will release fat stores. Hope this helps and here's to a wetter lifestyle…

CHAPTER 5

The Amazing World of Fats

This is not a lecture on weight management or obesity. I will take that on in a whole separate chapter later. I wanted to address inflammation in this chapter and realize it takes a basic knowledge of fats to understand what I am going to tell you about inflammation. Let's get the cart before the horse and talk about fats, a very complicated and controversial topic in the world of health and nutrition.

Every day, literally, I read a new study which directly contradicts earlier studies on fats. You might be doing this, too. It is no wonder everyone is confused on this subject. Even people who spend their whole lives as scientists researching this topic cannot agree with each other. Basically, science has a long way to go to be able to broadcast a common and unified message about fats to help us know exactly what to consume in terms of good fats (Yes, there are good fats.) and what to avoid in terms of bad fats, not to mention the correct amount of fat to retain in our daily diets vs. other macronutrients like proteins and carbs.

Remember when you read articles/studies about fats this and fats that, if the article does not tell you what kind of fat was used and how it was prepared, then the information is worthless, because all fats are not created equal.

But there is some common and unified knowledge I feel comfortable in sharing about fats that may help lower the confusion bar. The number one thing is that all 40 trillion (give or take 10 trillion, no one really knows) or so cells in our body are surrounded by a cell wall and the main component of that wall is fat. In one model of health, called the Barrier Model (my term), our health is controlled by regulation of substances flowing across various barriers in our body; everything from our emotional barriers to our digestive, circulatory, brain and cellular barriers.

On the cellular level, our cell functions are protected through a flow/prevention of nutrients/toxins between the outer cellular environment and the inner cellular environment; a very tightly controlled flow, second by second, of what comes into a cell and what leaves the cell. And the story does not stop there.

There is also a double fat wall around the mitochondria (our energy factories) in each cell and a fat wall around our nucleus (within each cell) that contains our DNA. In each case, these fat or lipid bilayers (barriers) all serve the same purpose, a protective barrier that enables proper cell/organelle function. When these semi-permeable fat barriers don't work right, cells don't work right and you get diseases. It is that simple.

Controlling your fat intake to only good fats your body needs for proper cell barrier function is one of the great health keys to a happy body.

But let's back up a bit. As I said, all fats are not created equal. Let's get into a bit of detail here. You can put fats into four basic categories: saturated, mono unsaturated, poly unsaturated and trans fats, depending on how many hydrogen atoms are attached to the fat molecule (which is essentially a long series of carbon atoms linked together in a chain with hydrogen atoms hanging on). We are a carbon-based life form! If all the hydrogen atoms are present and accounted for (a military term ☺), then you have a saturated fat (fully saturated with hydrogen). Mono unsaturated means it is missing one hydrogen atom. Poly unsaturated means it is missing more than one hydrogen atom. A trans-fat is an unsaturated fat (missing one or more hydrogen atoms) where at least one hydrogen atom is on the opposite side of the molecule across a carbon to carbon-double bond.

Some, but not many, trans fats occur naturally but are mainly manufactured (synthetic) by humans trying to sell us unhealthy products. The trans-fat configuration makes the fat molecule straight, vs. the normal or "Sis" configuration (hydrogens on the same side) in an unsaturated fat, making the molecule bend (normally what you want in an unsaturated fat). The saturated fats and the trans fats are mostly solid at room temperature. (This is why companies make trans fats. They take cheap runny oil, change their structure, add flavoring, and Voilà! You have artificial butter, for example!)

The bottom line here is that trans fats are fake, manmade saturated fats, with a changed fat structure and do not perform well for your body. Don't forget, at any given time, your cell will 'plug and play' different fats into your cell wall to get different transportation of different nutrients/toxins across the cell membrane (wall).

Our body can make many of its own fats. But there are some fats our bodies cannot make, these are *essential fatty acids*. You must bring these in through your diet. Now you are probably asking, "What are the essential fatty acids?" There are only two: Omega 3s and Omega 6s. They are both poly unsaturated fatty acids, meaning they are missing more than one hydrogen atom in their carbon chain structure. The 3 or 6 simply means the point on the carbon chain where the missing hydrogen atoms start, either the 3rd carbon from the end or the 6th carbon from the end.

These two fats, and all the fats in your body that are made from these two, must be in the right form and structure so that when your cells reach out and grab them and insert them into your cell walls, they can perform as nature intended. Otherwise, your cells will not function correctly, and disease will follow.

One more thing, fat can also be used as a fuel. You can burn glucose, you can burn protein (after having been converted to glucose) or you can burn fat. Depending on your genetics and other factors, some people are better fat burners than others. And, we won't get into sports physiology and how the body decides what to burn at any given time. Just know that fat can be a very important energy source for you at the right time, when your body needs it, a key understanding in weight loss strategies as well, which I already told you, I will get into in a different chapter.

All of this is to say that it is critical in overall health management to have only good fats in your body, so your cells and energy systems work at peak efficiency. Just like a car, bad oil (fats), over time, will bring you to a screeching halt. Think of it like this: America is in need of an oil (fats) change!!

What makes a fat bad? Air, heat, light or altering its structure through man-made fats such as hydrogenation (creation of trans fats). Some fats are very stable at room temperature and do not go rancid easily such as coconut oil that is mainly different varieties of saturated fat. Other fats go bad in 15 minutes at room temperature like flax seed oil, mostly poly unsaturated fat which is high in Omega 3. All vegetable oils you buy in the store are rancid and oxidized (causing inflammation) unless they are cold processed and kept in the fridge and away from light and open air. One exception is extra virgin organic olive oil (EVOOO) which has naturally occurring plant compounds that fight rancidity at room temperature.

You don't notice the rancidity in commercial oils because they add a perfume and flavorings to the oil to disguise how bad it tastes and smells. The manufactured fats (trans fats) are a different chemical structure and therefore a different physical form, and form is very important in performance in cell membranes (walls). So those trans fats will disrupt the ability of your cells to regulate internal cellular environments.

Heating fats destroys them by altering structure. So, all commercially fried food which is fried in vegetable oil (unsaturated fat) are super-heated and are bad for you. If you must fry food, do it at home in saturated fat (higher smoke point) like high quality, grass fed Lard (preferably with no pesticides, no antibiotics, low Omega 6s (grain fed animals are high in Omega 6), coconut oil or grass-fed butter.

Different fats have different smoke points for cooking so if you stay below the smoke point, you will get better quality fats. I only use coconut oil or butter for cooking because they are mainly saturated fat and therefore more stable at the higher cooking temperatures. Extra virgin organic olive oil is good, but I just use it directly on my salads/organic popcorn/etc. without heating because it has a low smoke point. (There is still debate in the natural health world on olive oil, even if cold processed although the evidence is mounting that it has extremely good benefits for the body and brain.)

A Mediterranean diet is loaded with olive oil and has been shown to be a vast improvement over a typical western diet. But some purists claim that is due to the increase in beans and nuts and olives, not the oil. I have seen at least one well-done study directly showing the benefits of olive oil on the body.

Nature has provided the perfect way to consume vegetable/seed fats (oils) in that nature protects them from light and air by encapsulating them in protective seed/fruit coatings and combines them with plant compounds. A great way to get your plant-based Omega 3s is through flax/chia seeds or cold pressed and refrigerated organic flax oil in opaque bottles. If you eat flax seeds, you must grind flax seeds right before consumption due to the thick shell surrounding the seeds (nature's way of protecting the oil) that prevent absorption of the oil. Or, you can grind enough for about one week and keep it in the freezer. This is also a great source of fiber and an aid to estrogen/testosterone control. Other good sources of Omega 3s are animal Omega 3s from salmon and sardines, or properly treated (cold processed) krill oil. I recommend a balance of plant-based Omega 3s and animal-based Omega 3s (they are different). We will get into the right balance of Omega 3s and Omega 6s in a future chapter when we start talking about inflammation, the number one cause of disease in the U.S. today.

Other sources of good fats are organic: raw nuts (not peanuts), seeds, avocados, Ghee (butter with casein removed), raw nut butters, properly processed fish oils and supplements, grass fed butter, and virgin coconut oil.

There is much debate on how much saturated fat (butter/eggs/coconut/lard/beef fat) to include in your diet so until there is clarity and agreement from science, I am not going to address this. But I can say that Medium Chain Triglycerides (MCTs) oils (mainly in coconut oils) have been absolute life savers to people with various brain disorders because MCTs are quickly broken down to ketone bodies and your brain cells can burn ketone bodies as energy very easily. Also, the main ketones, Beta Hydroxy Butyrate and Acetoacetate, have also proven to be highly anti-inflammatory, improve gene expression, improve immune function and prevent lean muscle loss and thus have shown utility in cancer treatment and prevention in non-human experiments.

There are many studies going on in labs around the world now looking at the benefits of moving into a state of ketosis where your body is using primarily ketones from fats for energy.

There is a wealth of topics I could talk about here, including the effects of fat (some positive, some negative) on cholesterol/obesity/ intestinal permeability/allergies/autoimmunity/ nerve function and heart disease, but this is meant as simply a primer for the chapter on inflammation.

Here is an excerpt from one of Dr. Mark Hyman's articles, one of the foremost medical doctors working to unscramble the differing science research results on fat. The article discusses common health Myths. Here is his Myth #4 which deals with fats:

MYTH #4
FAT MAKES YOU FAT

Here's another pet peeve of mine: the notion that eating fat makes you fat. Fat is not a four-letter word! Eating fat not only doesn't make you fat, it's critical to health and weight loss. Studies comparing a high-fat diet that is identical in calorie count to a high-sugar diet had totally different effects on metabolism. The higher-fat diet caused people to burn an extra 300 calories a day. That's the equivalent of running for an hour without doing any exercise.

Dietary fat actually speeds up your metabolism, while sugar slows it down. The right kinds of fat cool down inflammation, while sugar fuels it.

In studies of animals that ate identical calorie diets of either low-fat (high-sugar) or higher-fat and protein diets showed that higher-sugar diets led to more fat deposition and muscle loss, while the higher-fat and protein diets led to more muscle mass and fat loss. Keep in mind they were eating exactly the same number of calories.

The right fats are actually your cells' preferred fuel, especially those fats called medium-chain triglycerides (MCTs) that come from foods like coconut oil and coconut butter.

Yes, stay away from trans fats, but good fats like extra-virgin olive oil, coconut butter, avocado, nuts, seeds and nut butters keep us full and lubricate the wheels of our metabolism. Please stop fearing fat!"

Just remember most all good fats are good for most people and bad fats are bad for everyone. The jury is still out on saturated fats, possibly because there are many different types of saturated fats and we are learning that some are good for you and some can be damaging. I apologize for the technical detail in this article, but I know of no other way to get you started in understanding all the stuff you see out there in the mysterious world of fats.

I must recognize the great work from Doctors Dean Ornish and Caldwell Esselstyn who both have cured cardiovascular disease (CVD) by putting patients on plant-based diets, taking them off of dairy, meat, fish, oils, sugary foods and drinks and processed foods. The evidence is clear and unambiguous. I would highly advise anyone with CVD to look into these doctors and follow their protocols.

From this strong evidence, I reason that plant-based fats are good for you, if protected from oxidation/rancidity/structure change, that is, from heat, air and light. Your body needs essential fatty acids but keep your system free of harmful oils. Anytime you buy all those cooking oils at the store, you are asking for trouble. Cook with more stable coconut oil or lower heated grass-fed butter. Don't overcook your meats and eat them sparingly. Use MCTs to get you into ketosis, if you want to try that. Keep your flax oil/seed cold. Stay tuned to the science. Maybe someday, we will hear a consistent message about fats.

CHAPTER 6

The Problem with Sugar

The human body controls levels of sugar in your bloodstream very tightly to around five grams or one teaspoon at any given time because too little or too much results in permanent damage or death.

The average American consumes 22 teaspoons of sugar a day!

Our hormonal control systems were never designed to handle fast changes in blood sugar levels. These hormonal controls work best with gentle rises and falls in blood sugar. That is why all-natural sugar comes with complex (unprocessed), not simple (processed) sugars that are combined with fat and/or fiber or complexity (multiple sugar molecules joined together), to slow conversion (absorption) of sugar into the bloodstream.

Why make your body work so hard all the time in over using hormone control mechanisms to keep your sugar levels under control? This is energy you could be using for other essential processes. Simple processed (refined) sugars (including white flours) are at the root of most chronic disease today, not only due to the below conditions listed, but because they are empty calories, fooling you into thinking you are giving your body the nutrition it needs, when in fact your body is crying out due to starvation from a lack of essential fatty acids, amino acids, vitamins, minerals and polyphenols (plant nutrients).

When I think of sugar, I think of three things: manipulation, addiction and starvation in a loop of functionality. Manipulation from the food scientists hired by Big Food to manipulate you into buying their product with known addictive substances: addiction from sugar that stimulates similar neural pathways as heroin.

Starvation in that you are literally starving your body (ever so slowly) to death. In a state of starvation, your body tells you to eat more, but it does not have the ability to tell you it needs this or that vitamin or mineral, just that it is starving. Thus, being fooled by Big Food, you turn to more empty calories, your heroin addiction of choice…sugar. Once again, the body is not designed to deal with pure sugar. Do you see any sugar seeds growing on plants anywhere?

Here are some of the issues with excessive and sudden sugar spikes:

- Brain: can rewire the brain's pathways. Diets full of processed and sugar-heavy foods (high glycemic) can increase the risk of depression by 58%.
- Skin: Proteins incorporate sugar as part of their structure, aging skin and causing wrinkles.
- Genitals: Excess sugar can impair blood flow, upping the risk of erectile dysfunction in men and sexual arousal disorder in women.
- Heart: Sugar inflames the linings of the arteries to the heart, increasing the risk of stroke and heart attack.
- Diabetes: Excess sugar causes insulin spikes which causes insulin resistance at the cellular level and pancreas exhaustion leading to Type 2 diabetes.

- Kidneys: Sugar overload can damage the kidney filtration system. Diabetes is one of the main causes of kidney failure.
- Joints: High sugar diets pump inflammatory compounds into your bloodstream, which can increase arthritis pain and joint damage.
- Weight Gain: Excess sugar spikes insulin which, in order to protect the body from sugar damage, converts sugar to fat, increasing body weight and preventing fat loss.
- Pathogenic Bacteria: Sugar feeds the wrong bacteria in your gut, which secrete toxins into your blood stream and crowd out your good bacteria, short changing you on all sorts of critical fatty acids and vitamins they are providing, and further adding to your weight gain problems. Many studies have shown stubborn weight loss issues are related to bad gut microbial populations.
- Candida Infections: Candida feeds off sugar. These infections can drain you of your energy, eating all of the sugar in your blood and leaving you with not enough to power your cells.
- Cancer: Cancer loves sugar. A cancer cell uses mainly anaerobic fermentation (without oxygen) producing only 3-4 molecules of ATP (our energy molecule) per molecule of sugar versus a normal cell which produces 43 molecules of ATP. Thus, in order to survive, it must hog all the sugar in your blood. That is why cancer patients are so weak. No sugar is left to power your normal cells. Stop the sugar, starve your cancer cells.
- Endocrine Organ Fatigue: Our endocrine (hormonal) organs maintain blood sugar levels in a very tight

dance and feedback loop. They were not meant to be constantly jerked around, trying to respond to drastic changes in sugar levels with all the snacks, candy, sodas and meals of processed sugars. This leads to adrenal and pancreas exhaustion and cellular hormonal resistance.

- Alzheimer's: Some of the latest research on Alzheimer's reveals that those effected with the disease have insulin resistance in your brain cells, preventing uptake of sugar and therefore needed fuel for brain energy production. Insulin resistance, as mentioned before is caused by over production of insulin, which is caused by constantly exceeding and spiking blood sugar levels. Some have called this Diabetes type 3.
- Nerve Damage: High sugar levels damage nerves over time, as all diabetics know. "High blood sugar is toxic to your nerves," says pain management specialist Robert Bolash, MD. "When a nerve is damaged, you may feel tingling, pins and needles, burning or sharp, stabbing pain." Numbness in the feet can lead to undetected infections and amputations.
- Addiction: Simple sugars stimulate the same neural pathways as does heroin. You literally need more and more to get the same result. There are ways to break this addiction. Please see me if you are interested.
- Minerals: Excess sugar can disrupt the balance of essential minerals in your body. It can even lead to the depletion of your stored minerals. One good example of this can be seen with the mineral Calcium. Studies have shown that sugar increases the rate of calcium excretion. This can throw off the calcium-magnesium

ratio and the calcium-phosphorus ratio that your body needs.

- Allergies/Chronic Infection: Sugar can lead to food allergies. Digestion requires that your food get broken down into its essential parts. This takes place because of the function of enzymes. Eating excess sugar can mess up the balance of essential minerals (as seen above) and that can mess up the function of enzymes which digest your food. Thus, undigested food can enter your blood stream and cause allergies keeping your immune system on constant high alert, exhausting your immunity and setting you up for chronic infection.
- Weakened Immune System: Loma Linda University did a study on sugar intake and phagocytes (part of your immune system). In the study it was shown that these phagocytes decreased their consumption of invaders dramatically for up to six hours after eating sugar. This is bad news for fighting infections and cancer.

But along with sugar, there are direct problems from the higher insulin levels caused by the sugar spikes. I suspect as the science becomes clearer, we will see that the main problem here is higher insulin levels that precede sugar issues and cause sugar metabolism issues. Here are known problems caused directly from high insulin levels (caused by sugar spikes):

✓ Excess insulin remaining in the blood after a meal has been identified as a major cause of nonalcoholic fatty liver disease.

✓ Hyperinsulinemia is an independent risk factor for kidney disease among metabolic syndrome patients.

- ✓ High insulin blood levels are predictive of Type II diabetes and strongly associated with obesity.

- ✓ In a study on variables that are associated with Alzheimer's, the number one association was with a particular gene called ApoA4. Number two was, drum roll please...high insulin levels. Number three was age. That is a shocker! That means you can get Alzheimer's at any age with the wrong diet and lifestyle choices (over consumption of carbs and sugar).

- ✓ A number of published studies indicate that high insulin levels drive the development and progression of many types of malignancies.

I know it can be tough to reduce sugar in your routines. And, many of the sugar alternatives are downright toxic, destroy your gut microbiome and keep you from losing weight. I have found Stevia and Monk Fruit are the best so far because they are natural plant extracts, unprocessed and do not spike blood sugar levels.

Hope this was not sugar overload for you and that you can move into a more sugar-free lifestyle.

THOUGHT BREAK #2: ROOT CAUSE PHILOSOPHY

Through years of pondering the root cause of disease, I have come to believe it comes down to four things: emotional state, physical toxicity, nutritional deficiency and aging, and of course, in our system of systems, these are all related.

It is important to get to the root cause rather than just treat the symptom. Don't get me wrong, treating the symptom can be a very important temporary fix to get you out of pain and discomfort, and give your body time to recover, but it is usually not curative, and could bind you to a permanent drug or compound that has side effects, which over the long-term causes damage. And remember, drugs and medical treatment kill hundreds of thousands every year. So, if at all possible, it is better to treat the cause of the disease or do both symptom treatment and cause treatment at the same time, so you can eventually get off of the symptom stuff.

Now, people are basically lazy and resist change. This is not an indictment, just my observation. They don't want to change anything in their lives for many reasons, so treating the symptom is much easier than making the changes it takes to treat the cause.

Many of you reading this will want to consider taking baby steps – small, slow and steady alterations, moving towards a healthier you. There is some argument for this in terms of body healing. Most likely, it took many years of poor habits to result in symptoms. Look at the case of auto-immunity. We know now that increased levels of tissue antibodies that show the beginnings of auto immunity occur years before the onset of symptoms. Cancer is the same way. Taking years to develop and kill you. This is your body's way of contributing to the preservation of the species, to get you through your prime reproductive years. So, we cannot expect to heal instantly either. Taking baby steps, doing something, just one new thing each week, or month, is kind of at a pace to give the body a chance to adjust and heal at its pace as well. (See my Laws of Life page 21).

There is nothing you can do to speed up the body. All you can do is address the three and sometimes four (see the chapter on anti-aging strategies) root causes, and then stand back and let the magic happen, the magic of the prime drive of creation; self-preservation and self-healing.

It is interesting how medical science has gone the opposite way, away from simplification and into complexity when physics and chemistry have always searched for simplicity and theories of unification. Physics is now down to a few unifying theories, and physicists are hard at work proving a single root organizing principle behind all physical laws at the subatomic level. Chemistry has a unifying periodic table of elements, having discovered the underlying principle on how elements are organized and found.

Why isn't medical science hard at work to determine the single unifying cause of disease? Instead, you have to see four or five doctors to get to your issue, because of diversification and complexity in the medical field.

We need root cause medicine, not as alternative medicine as it is now, but as a mainstream primary form of treatment. Surprisingly, we seem to be moving in that direction.

CHAPTER 7

Get Your Proteins Right

When I think of protein, here is what comes to mind: The breakdown of dietary protein into smaller segments called peptides and then one step further into individual amino acids, then absorption through our intestinal walls into our blood and lymph, transport to our cells and then reconstruction back into the proteins that our body needs (under the direction of our DNA) in order to do a million functions in the body.

I think of acid reflux which causes most people to take acid blockers, which over time causes a reduced ability to break down proteins into amino acids that your body so desperately needs (you have to have acid to activate the digestive enzymes that breakdown protein in the stomach).

I think of leaky gut syndrome where undigested proteins get absorbed into the blood and lymph and cause adverse immune reactions leading to allergies, autoimmune disease and weight gain.

I think of lean muscle mass and where the right balance is between strength/protein ingestion and length of life (explained later), especially as we get older when there is a natural loss of muscle over time.

I think of the continual recycling of our own body protein forming a constant supply for us to draw upon, as we destroy old cells and create new ones, thus lowering our requirement for dietary protein.

I think of pH balance where too much acidity in the blood (mainly from too much meat protein) causes the body to break down muscle mass to balance our blood pH, rather than gain muscle mass as the right amount of protein will produce, or cause osteoporosis when the body pulls calcium out of the bones to balance our pH.

I think of questions like, "How much protein do I need on a daily basis to stay healthy, and what are my best sources of protein? Do I need a dense source of protein (animal-based) for every meal? Are there essential amino acids the body must consume because we cannot manufacture them ourselves, and where is the dividing line where too much protein becomes dangerous? And, can a vegetarian diet be healthy over the long term?"

I will attempt to chip away at these issues by sharing some of the latest science on proteins, so you can make your own decisions.

In general: Do you need dietary protein? Yes, absolutely.

Can too much of the wrong protein be dangerous? Yes.

Is everyone different on their protein needs? To a point...Yes. We all need a minimum amount, then it varies from there.

Are there different types and qualities of protein? Yes.

Is there some protein in everything we eat, including vegetables and fruit? Yes.

Can the body make its own protein from its in-house amino acid pool? Yes.

Do we dump, reabsorb and reuse protein every day in our digestive tract? Yes.

Do we need dense protein (animal-based) at every meal? No.

Are there some people who can be successful vegetarians and others who cannot? Yes, but this requires more study to figure out the genetics involved. Plus, to be a successful vegetarian takes knowledge and work to do it right to insure you are getting the essential nutrition your body needs.

Is there a link between protein and muscle mass? Yes. But protein is not the only consideration here. Muscle mass is also a function of testosterone levels, so both must be optimum to gain muscle (By the way, did you know that testosterone is made from cholesterol?)

And, one other factor in maintaining and growing muscle is overall calorie intake. You cannot gain muscle if your body is low in calories because your body in a chronic low-calorie state will go to your muscle and start using that for a fuel source causing muscle wasting. So, as you will see below, you must make a decision here, because calorie restriction (CR) activates genetic repair and extends lifespan.

The trick is to find the right balance
between adequate strength and restricted calories.

Is there a trade-off between long life at moderate strength and a shorter life with super muscles? Yes.

As we age, do we lose muscle mass and therefore have to adjust our protein and work outs to stay at the same level of strength? Yes.

Is there a link between digestive/intestinal health and protein assimilation? Yes.

Is there a link between body acidity, protein and bone mass/kidney health/gout? Yes. Too much protein, through metabolism, acidifies the body. To bring pH back into balance, the body draws minerals from the bones and nitrogen from muscle tissue leading to bone density problems and muscle reduction.

Added nitrogen in the blood turns into ammonia and crystals putting a strain on the kidneys and creating gout problems.

Is there a link between Sulphur-bearing protein and health? Yes. Sulphur-bearing amino acids are critical to our health in many ways.

Are there essential amino acids that you must get through food that the body cannot make by itself? Yes.

Do you need all essential amino acids at every meal? No.

Can too much protein contribute to diabetes? Yes. A portion of all the protein you eat is converted into glucose for fuel, thus you can spike your blood sugar and insulin levels leading to diabetes issues.

Any more questions? Nope. That's it. The end. Just kidding.

The New Science of Trimethylamine Oxide (TMAO)

TMA or tryimethylamine is produced by certain bacteria in the gut when fed choline or carnitine which are found in red meat and eggs. The TMA travels to your liver which then adds the O or oxide. The TMAO causes buildup of cholesterol on the arteries and thus, heart attacks. So, the more red meat or eggs you have, the more gut bacteria you build up that can turn those compounds into TMA. In the case of meat or carnitine, there is a clear link to heart disease.

However, in the case of egg yolks (a good source of choline), we know they can be very heart protective. Something in eggs is countering the effect of the TMAO levels and this still needs to be studied (Could it be the high Sulphur content since we know Sulphur is critical to our health?).

Also, in meat, as mentioned above, protein metabolic byproducts acidify the blood and can cause crystal formation causing gout. Body balancing mechanisms react to the higher acid levels by buffering with minerals, namely calcium.

Unfortunately, the calcium comes from the bones, thus leading to bone density issues. Plus, when certain types of protein like casein from milk are taken in excess, it has been shown to be carcinogenic.

There are two proteins in milk: casein and whey. If you are supplementing with casein, move to whey and lower your consumption of cow milk. Also, whey is excellent for stimulating our inborn antioxidant production called glutathione, which is critical to mitigating the negative effects (waste products) of glucose metabolism, namely Reactive Oxygen Species, very destructive oxidants to your body.

It appears we don't all have the same bacteria in our guts. What we do have is dictated by our dietary patterns, pointed out Dr. Hazen in a Cleveland Clinic news release:

"A diet high in carnitine (from meat) actually shifts our gut microbe composition to those that like carnitine, making meat eaters even more susceptible to forming TMAO and its artery-clogging effects. Meanwhile, vegans and vegetarians have a significantly reduced capacity to synthesize TMAO from carnitine."

How much red meat is too much?

An important question this new study does not answer is: Can we eat very small amounts of lean red meat (no more than 4 ounces weekly, as the Pritikin Eating Plan recommends), and still have, like the vegetarians and vegans studied, gut bacteria that keep TMAO production down?

"We just don't know what amount of red meat is low enough to look like the long-term vegetarian and vegans studied," Dr. Hazen told *Pritikin Perspective*. He himself still eats steak "but much less frequently" – no more than twice a month, and in much smaller portions, about four to six ounces.

"Odds are the bacteria that induce TMAO production from dietary carnitine would largely die off on an eating plan like Pritikin," surmises Dr. Kenney. "And so, the occasional lean red meat meal would likely result in very little TMAO getting produced."

Now, let's cover the mTOR or mammalian Target of Rapamycin pathway. I know it is a mouthful, but you need to know about it. This pathway is a nutrition sensor (not just protein but all fuel sources: protein, carbs and fats) and signaling pathway. When it is upregulated, it stimulates growth. When it is down regulated, it stimulates repair. Unfortunately, you cannot have it both ways. So, if you are always in the growth phase, you will not be able to keep up with all the damage that naturally occurs during the course of your lifetime, thus shortening lifespan.

If you want to expand your lifespan, you will have to have nutritional rest, to enter the repair cycles of your body. Your body is in a constant state of activity which creates DNA, soft tissue and muscle damage, creating a need for constant repair.

When breakdown exceeds repair capabilities, accelerated aging occurs. Obese people are at an extra disadvantage because not only are they not getting nutritional rest, but the weight alone puts their joints in an increased rate of tear down, exceeding the body's repair capabilities, thus leading to destroyed joints.

The mTOR pathway is one reason why fasting can be so healthful to the body.

Almost all religions of the world advocate some type of fasting regimen, some more than others. It is interesting that the folks studied for the Mediterranean diet and the long-lived people of Crete, do regular fasting to some degree one to two days a week, specifically avoiding meat for those days, but these facts have never come out as to why they enjoy good health and longevity. There is also a National Geographic study of what is called Blue Zones, those zones around the world where people live the longest.

The two things they found common to those zones are that people get exercise as part of their normal daily routines, and that they all have high consumptions of beans, interestingly enough. So, excessive proteins can keep you in the growth phase, keeping mTOR upregulated, and keep repair functions suppressed.

In one 2014 study involving more than 6,380 American adults over the age of 50, those who ate a diet high in animal protein:

- Had a 75% increase in overall mortality over the course of 18 years.
- Were 400% more likely to die of cancer than those who restricted their animal protein. (According to the authors, this association vanished when the protein was derived from plants.)
- Had a 500% increase in diabetes across all ages.

The only people who benefited from a high-protein diet were seniors over the age of 65. In this age group, high amounts of animal protein were associated with reduced cancer and overall mortality risk. According to the authors:

"These results suggest that low protein intake during middle age followed by moderate- to high-protein consumption in old adults may optimize health span and longevity."

Let's talk about sulphur-bearing protein. This is an important aspect of consuming protein because we want to make sure we get adequate amounts of sulphur in our diet. Sulphur is critical to proper liver function (detoxification of chemicals, toxic waste, drugs, alcohol, etc.) and many other functions in the body, many of which are still under intensive scientific investigation.

Methionine is not only an amino acid-bearing sulphur, but is also critical to methylation and epigenetics, discussed in other chapters. Methionine from dietary protein is also critical to producing glutathione, one the most important antioxidants in your body.

Protein foods that contain the sulfur have the sulphur-bearing amino acids methionine, cystine and cysteine. Eggs are among the highest dietary sources of sulfur, with meat, poultry and fish also providing large amounts. For vegans and vegetarians, non-GMO soy products and other legumes are good sources of the sulfur-containing amino acids. Interesting that legumes (beans) are also one of the common foods in the Blue Zones discussed above. Nuts, seeds and grains are also good vegetarian sources of methionine. I personally supplement with one teaspoon of MSM five days a week to ensure I am getting enough sulphur in my diet.

Maybe one more caution about too much meat. Of course, we all know that animals are meant to eat grass and bugs – not grains, hormones, pesticides, herbicides, GMOs and gosh knows what else they feed them that pass on to us as we eat them. We also have found a correlation (not causation) between too high meat consumption and high estrogen levels in the body. For women, this means increased risk for breast cancer and obesity. For men, this means increased risk for prostate cancer and obesity. Remember, correlation does not equal causation, but the correlation is there.

Now, on the other hand, too little protein can be devastating as well. Vegetarians must be very careful about protein intake to make sure they are getting enough in quantity and that they are covering all eight essential amino acids by varying food intake. If you are vegetarian, look below for the eight essential amino acids and then the foods that contain all eight and make sure and include those in your eating routine along with sufficient amount of protein for your daily requirements.

Here is more interesting information on protein. **Not all** the amino acids from protein get turned into proteins in your body. Some of them are turned into glucose and are burned for energy as mentioned earlier.

This is a remnant of our caveman days. When we were cavemen, food was scarce. So, we needed to be able to get energy regardless of what food we ate.

Berries? No problem. They contain carbs that are burned for energy. Nuts? They contain fats that are burned for energy. Freshly killed squirrel? Some of the protein in the meat is turned into lean body mass, and the rest of it is turned into glucose for energy.

So, how can you tell if your body is using the protein for muscle or if it's turning it into excess glucose? Scientists have answered this question. You see, amino acids contain nitrogen. And when amino acids are turned into proteins, the nitrogen remains in your body as part of the protein. But when amino acids are converted into sugar, the nitrogen is released and passes through to your urine.

So, if you want to know if your food is being turned into protein or sugar, all you do is measure the amount of nitrogen in your urine! This measurement is called Amino Acid Utilization, or AAU. Here's how it works:

If a dietary protein has an AAU of 100%, it means that there is no nitrogen in your urine and that the body is using 100% of the amino acids in that food to build body protein. That's great!

On the other hand, if a protein source has an AAU of 10% that means your body is only using 10% of the amino acids to make body protein. That means your body is turning 90% of those amino acids into sugar. Not good!

So, what's the best source of dietary protein, with the highest AAU? Scientists found that it's breast milk, with an AAU of 49%. That makes sense, because babies need an efficient source of dietary protein. But we're not babies, so what's the next best source of protein?

The next best source of protein is whole eggs. Whole eggs have an AAU of 47%. But, it has to be the whole egg. If you eat egg whites like many so-called health experts tell you to do, you will only get an AAU of 17%. Why? Because egg yolks contain the essential amino acid methionine. Take out the yolk, and you seriously limit the egg's protein-building value.

After whole eggs come meat, poultry, and fish. They're all equal, with an AAU of 32%. But it really goes downhill from there.

So, let's go back to the original problem. Why do people lose so much lean body mass as they get older? There are three main reasons (these insights are from Dr. Shallenberger):

The first reason is that they're not eating enough protein. The second is that they are eating the wrong sources of protein. And the third is that they are not digesting their protein. You see, it's not enough to eat the right proteins; you also have to digest those proteins and break them down into amino acids.

Unfortunately, the older we get, the weaker our digestive systems tend to be. We make less stomach acid and digestive enzymes. And this can cause a downward spiral.

Remember earlier when I mentioned that enzymes are actually proteins? Well, if you're protein-deficient, it stands to reason that you would not make enough digestive enzymes. That means that you would not digest your food properly. This would make you even more protein-deficient which would lead to even lower enzyme production. And so on.

What if you didn't have to rely on your digestive system to break down protein? What if you could skip that part of the process entirely and just take amino acids? The amino acids would go directly into your bloodstream. They would then be used to build **muscle, bone, connective tissue, hormones, enzymes, and more.**

So that is one strategy as you get older, supplement with straight essential amino acids. There are many such products on the market that can ensure you get all eight essential amino acids, those acids your body cannot make itself (L-Leucine, L-Valine, L-Isoleucine, L-Lysine HCI, L-Phenylalanine, L-Threonine, L-Methionine, L-Tryptophan). One of the supplementation products that looks good to me is from Advanced Bionutritionals that claims a UUA score of 99%. That is pretty impressive if it is true. Check for other possible supplement choices as you get older.

Keep in mind that your body goes into a self-cleaning mode called autophagy when there is a lack of protein and carbs in your system. This is a good thing. It is as if we were meant to have periods of low protein in our normal eating protocol. So, many folks are starting to cycle protein and carbs and enter periods of fasting called intermittent fasting. On those days, you could skip breakfast or just have a little fat in your hot drink, enough to get you through to lunch time, with a nice 16-hour fast, plenty of time to kick in self-cleaning. That way, you would get the advantage of cleaning on one day, then large protein and carb consumption on the other days. If you did this every other day, you would be getting the best of both worlds.

NINE SIGNS FROM DR.AXE YOU MAY NOT BE GETTING ENOUGH PROTEIN

1. **You have high cholesterol.** High cholesterol and triglycerides are not just caused by eating fatty foods — they are also a result of increased inflammation, hormonal imbalances and high-processed/high-sugar diets. If you tend to replace protein foods with sugary snacks, refined carbs and packaged convenient goods, your cholesterol can start to rise as your liver and cells process fats less efficiently. Some studies have even found an inverse relationship exists between protein intake and risk of heart disease.

2. **You're feeling more anxious and moodier.** Amino acids are the building blocks for neurotransmitters which control your mood. Proteins help the brain synthesize hormones like dopamine and serotonin that help bring on positive feelings like calm, excitement and positivity.

3. **Your workouts are suffering.** You're probably already aware that protein is needed to build new muscle mass, but it's also important for sustaining your energy and motivation. A low protein diet can result in muscle wasting (or muscle atrophy), fatigue and even fat gain — it can also be behind female athlete triad. In fact, you can work out more, but see less results if your diet isn't adequate to support tissue repair or your energy needs.

4. **You aren't sleeping well**. Poor sleep and insomnia can sometimes be linked to unstable blood sugar levels, a rise

in cortisol and a decrease in serotonin production. Blood sugar swings during the day carry over through the night. Carbohydrates require much more insulin than fat or protein does. Eating foods with protein before bed can help with tryptophan and serotonin production, and they have a minimal effect on blood glucose levels; in fact, protein slows down the absorption of sugar during a meal.

5. **You have "brain fog."** Protein is needed to support many aspects of healthy neurological functioning. Brain fog, poor concentration, lack of motivation and trouble learning new information can be signs that you're low in neurotransmitters you need to focus including dopamine, epinephrine, norepinephrine, and serotonin. Neurotransmitters are synthesized in the brain using amino acids, and studies show that balanced diets with enough protein can boost work performance, learning and motor skills

6. **You're gassy and can't go to the bathroom.** Many metabolic and digestive functions depend on amino acid intake. If your body feels fatigued and run down in general due to protein deficiency, enzyme production, muscle contractions in your GI tract and digestion in general will suffer.

7. **Your pants are feeling tighter.** Although sometimes higher in calories than carbs, high-protein foods cause increased satiety to a greater extent than carbohydrates or fats do, so they can prevent overeating and snacking. They also help stabilize your blood sugar, allow you to retain more muscle which burns more calories all day, and can reduce cravings.

8. **Your menstrual cycle is irregular.** One of the most common reasons women suffer from irregular periods and infertility is the condition known as polycystic ovary syndrome (PCOS). Two major risk factors for PCOS are obesity and pre-diabetes or diabetes — in fact, insulin resistance affects 50 to 70% of all women with PCOS. Low-protein, high-sugar/high-carb diets can contribute to insulin resistance, fatigue, inflammation and weight gain that disrupts the delicate balance of female hormones (including that of estrogen, progesterone and DHEA) needed to sustain a regular cycle.

9. **You've been getting injured more often and are slow to heal.** A low protein diet can raise your risk for muscle loss, falling, slow bone healing, bone weakness, fractures and even osteoporosis. Protein is needed for calcium absorption and helping with bone metabolism. Studies show that older adults with the greatest bone losses are those with a low protein intake of about 16 to 50 grams per day. Research also shows that a diet high in amino acids can help treat muscle loss due to aging (sarcopenia).

So, now the gorilla in the room: how much protein should we be getting? The Dietary Reference Intake (DRI) is .36 grams per pound of body weight. If you are a sedentary 140-pound person, you will need about 50 grams per day, although the number is slightly higher for men than it is for women. If you have a physically demanding job, you walk a lot, run, swim or do any sort of exercise, then you need more protein. Endurance athletes also need quite a bit of protein, about 0.5 – 0.65 grams per pound. Elderly people also need significantly more protein, up to 50% higher than the DRI, or about 0.45 to 0.6 grams per pound of bodyweight.

If your goal is to be a body builder, and accept the inherent risks of too much protein, then you can experiment to see what the right needs are to get the results you want. My advice is to stick to the minimum amount required to get those results and remember, there are some vegetarian body builders out there and large amounts of plant protein seem to be safer than large amounts of animal protein.

Since I have mentioned vegetarianism, I have known very successful vegetarians whose health is stellar, having been vegetarian for over 30 or more years. Many sects in India are vegetarian, some living well into their 100s. But then there are others who have damaged themselves by long-term vegetarianism. We don't have the studies that have closely monitored these two groups to see why some succeed and some fail.

Is it because of what they eat? There are hundreds of options while being vegetarian.

Are these unsuccessful ones eating high glycemic, low-protein vegetables?

Are they eating foods like wheat they are sensitive to? Are they primarily consuming processed foods and refined sugars, rancid oils and fats?

Are they getting sufficient micronutrients (vitamins and minerals and plant phytonutrients)?

Are they being careful to get a full complement of essential amino acids and fatty acids? Or, are they simply genetically different, making them incapable of utilizing the nutrients from vegetables as well as the successful vegetarian group? And conversely, if you are genetically capable, will eating meat make you less healthy? If so, how much and what kind of meat is good for you?

The answer is, we just don't know.

This is the field of nutrigenomics. Understanding what foods best work with your unique genetics can help you plan out and concentrate on those energy enhancing foods, providing a solid foundation for your body to heal, regain lost vitality, clear up allergies, lower inflammation and auto-immune issues, increase gut health and therefore nutrient absorption and result in reaching the correct weight for your body type. So, until the science is there, experiment. Go on a primarily plant-based diet as an initial step, eating salmon once or twice a week. See how you feel, listen to your body. Be a conscious eater, careful to get all the micronutrients your body needs. After several months, then you can move in one direction or the other, either going off meat entirely or slowly adding grass-fed meats or more of the smaller high omega-3 fish to your diet.

Then, check how you feel again. Keep making adjustments as you go. And your body changes with age, so change with it. Then you will see success for yourself.

One more word to the wise…macronutrient balance (protein vs. carbs vs. fats) is a very individual thing (n=1). Tons of macro studies have been done on thousands of people (n=hundreds or thousands) but what most functional nutritionist seem to be agreeing on now is (with the advancements in knowledge on epigenetics) everyone is different. Keep varying these ratios until you thrive, not survive, but thrive, without doing long-term damage to your connective tissue or that accelerates aging.

THOUGHT BREAK #3: IT'S A WILD RIDE

I was thinking about life in general, and it came to me that it's a pretty wild ride. "Like a roller coaster?" I asked myself. "No," I had to answer, "Far wilder than that."

You start off life at a fairly crazy speed. Think about it. The earth is revolving around itself at a thousand miles per hour, so you are moving immediately at a dizzying speed. Beyond that, the earth is moving at huge clip around the sun so not only are you hanging on going around and around, the whole tea cup (Oh, I hate that ride.) is going around a center point in a large circle. Of course, that is not where it ends.

The whole circle is moving in a giant spiral along with other solar systems towards the center of the galaxy, much like water going down a drain and if you are not sick yet, the whole galaxy is moving away at increasing speeds from the center of creation! Whew! Now that is a wild ride, more motion and at quicker speeds than you could ever get at a theme park.

So now you are supposed to conduct your life with these crazy pulls and motions going on, and perhaps most our lives are reflections of that – directions and motions so fast and so strong that sometimes all you can do is hang on for the ride. But there are points seemingly when I can make a decision and alter the course of the ride; which job to take, what sport to play, which car to drive, who to marry. But no matter which path I choose, overall, it still is a wild ride; whether I experience wealth, health and happiness or poverty, pain and struggle, whether I get married and have kids or get divorced or stay single.

Sometimes I think it is pretty wild to figure out why it is so wild. I am that I am. We are, and we are aware that we are. The constant quest to understand what it is all about, why are we here and what are we supposed to accomplish during our lifetimes.

Why do we live? Why do we die? Why do we suffer and why do we prosper? Why are some healthy and why are some sick? Is there a God and if so, who is she and how was she created? Why are there different languages and different skin colors and are we all basically the same? And if so, why are there wars, power struggles, different religions? It's enough to make you sick.

No wonder people sometimes just want to stop the ride, get off and take a breather before moving on. I guess we all should do that, forget about it all, get off the ride, take some quiet moments, change pace, relax, do something we enjoy, declare time our own.

Ignore the motions. Ignore the energy in motion (e-motions). Our great and mighty and complicated way of dealing with the world around us is still insufficient sometimes to deal with the ride without a clear and unambiguous break, at regular intervals. Otherwise, it is easy to get overwhelmed.

One thing is clear, some of the ride is out of our hands and to fight or resist those forces only serves to weaken us. I always have to remind myself to accept those things I cannot change, those forces greater than myself, and yet to keep on striving to improve things I can influence, as the Serenity Prayer says, "God, give me grace to accept with serenity the things that cannot be changed, courage to change the things which should be changed, and the wisdom to distinguish the one from the other." This is a difficult balance to achieve, by any stretch.

I can't help thinking that this ride never ends, that the physical life is merely another ride in the theme park of our spiritual journey. If that is true, I guess I need to understand this piece as it is and put it in context. Who knows, I might enjoy it more, lower stress, raise health and increase joy.

CHAPTER 8

Inflammation and Immunity

In previous chapters, we have covered a bit about hydration, the damaging effects of sugars and the basics on fats. Now, it's time we talk about inflammation. This is a long discussion because many things can cause inflammation, so I had to divide this discussion into two parts. Segment 2 will lay out more causes of inflammation plus some things you can do to help keep inflammation under control.

Some scientists believe that we can trace every single illness we have back to inflammation in the body somewhere. Others are more conservative in their assertions. I like to stay conservative until I see convincing scientific evidence from a majority of sources. So, in that vein, I divide illnesses into three categories when dealing with inflammation: 1) Known Inflammatory Diseases: like Asthma, Allergies, Rheumatoid Arthritis, Atopic Dermatitis, Gout, Lupus, Inflammatory Bowel Disease, Psoriasis, Scleroderma, Immuno Suppression 2) Diseases thought to be inflammation related: Atherosclerosis, Diabetes, Chronic Kidney Failure, Chronic Hepatitis, Chronic Thyroid Disease, Chronic Pancreatitis, Osteoarthritis, Chronic Bronchitis, Emphysema, Obesity, Other Auto Immune Conditions; 3) And those suspected to be caused by inflammation; like Cancer and Brain function disorders like Depression/ADHD/Memory loss/dementia.

This is a pretty impressive list, even being conservative. As a warning, this is no simple topic. There are mounds of deeply scientific research on this stuff. Don't get lost in detail (unless you want to!) So, what is inflammation you ask? Inflammation is a perfectly natural and healthy reaction of your immune system trying to protect and heal you.

For example, if you have an injury, the injury gets inflamed to send the right signals to bring in the biological and chemical troops in a series of steps to heal that injury. But like many control systems in your body, if left unchecked or if constantly over stimulated, it can have damaging consequences. Chronic (constant) stimulation of the immune system can lead to; the body not recognizing self, as in autoimmune conditions and therefore your body attacking itself, or to chronically inflamed areas where the immune system never shuts off, (it is supposed to shut down and pull the troops back to garrison when the battle has been won), that result in damaged organs, joints, and other tissues such as blood vessels. You can quickly see how perilous this situation can become.

So, what are the things that promote inflammation and keep the immune system over stimulated and what are the things that help to cool it down and keep it in proper balance or what we would call a state of homeostasis? Everything in the body, as in the universe, is about balance. Keep in mind a healthy immune system mobilizes an army of reactions, all with different functions, that are all supposed to pack up and go home once the battle has been won and your injury is healed, or infection is gone. If the troops stay on site and keep destroying things, that is where chronic damage from inflammation occurs.

So, let's talk about stress. Stress can cause chronic inflammation through too much cortisol production, a hormone produced by the adrenal gland. Through this mechanism, it can also cause adrenal fatigue, because if adrenals are always producing cortisol due to too much stress, then the gland will simply wear out, then you will be in real trouble with bouts of fatigue where you can hardly function throughout the day. But that is a different topic. Continuous stress causes high levels of cortisol in the system. Cortisol (as a steroid) functions to reduce inflammation in the body, which is good, but over time, these efforts to reduce inflammation also suppress the immune system, that is bad. Chronic suppression of the immune system leads to increased infections, an increased susceptibility to colds and other illnesses, an increased risk of cancer, the tendency to develop food allergies, an increased risk of an assortment of gastrointestinal issues (because a healthy intestine is dependent on a healthy immune system), and possibly an increased risk of autoimmune disease. All these illnesses all the time over stimulate the immune system leading to chronic inflammation.

Fats, as always are complicated. Rancid or oxidized fats (Unsaturated fats exposed to heat, light or air as mentioned before) are inflammatory. Also, human fat cells produce inflammatory messengers, so obese people are dealing with inflammatory conditions. MCT fats (mainly in coconut oil) on the other hand, are anti-inflammatory, so that is good. Also, getting the right balance of Omega 3s to Omega 6s is critical to getting inflammation under control. Here is a piece from Chris Kresser, a famous health practitioner, that covers this particular aspect of inflammation pretty well:

HOW TOO MUCH OMEGA-6 AND NOT ENOUGH OMEGA-3 IS MAKING US SICK

on MAY 8, 2010 by Chris Kresser

At the onset of the industrial revolution (about 140 years ago), there was a marked shift in the ratio of n-6 to n-3 fatty acids in the diet. Consumption of n-6 fats ***increased*** *at the expense of n-3 fats. This change was due to both the advent of the modern vegetable oil industry and the increased use of cereal grains as feed for domestic livestock (which in turn altered the fatty acid profile of meat that humans consumed). The following chart lists the Omega-6 and Omega-3 content of various vegetable oils and foods:*

Oil	Omega-6 Content	Omega-3 Content
Safflower	75%	0%
Sunflower	65%	0%
Corn	54%	0%
Cottonseed	50%	0%
Sesame	42%	0%
Peanut	32%	0%
Soybean	51%	7%
Canola	20%	9%
Walnut	52%	10%
Flaxseed	14%	57%
Fish*	0%	100%

Vegetable oil consumption rose dramatically between the beginning and end of the 20th century, and this had an entirely *predictable effect on the ratio of Omega-6 to Omega-3 fats in the American diet. Between 1935 and 1939, the ratio of n-6 to n-3 fatty acids **was reported** to be 8.4:1. From 1935 to 1985, this ratio increased to 10.3:1 (a 23% increase). Other calculations put the ratio as high as 12.4:1 in 1985. Today, estimates of the ratio range from an average of 10:1 to 20:1, with a ratio **as high as 25:1** in some individuals.*

In fact, Americans now get almost 20% of their calories from a single food source – soybean oil – with almost 9% of all calories from the Omega-6 fat linoleic acid (LA) alone!

This reveals that our average intake of n-6 fatty acids is between 10 and 25 times higher than evolutionary norms. The consequences of this dramatic shift cannot be overestimated.

Omega-6 competes with Omega-3, and vice versa

N-6 and n-3 fatty acids compete for the same conversion enzymes. This means that the quantity of n-6 in the diet directly affects the conversion of n-3 ALA, found in plant foods, to long-chain n-3 EPA and DHA, which protect us from disease.

*Several **studies** have shown that the biological availability and activity of n-6 fatty acids are inversely related to the concentration of n-3 fatty acids in tissue. Studies have also **shown** that greater composition of EPA & DHA in membranes reduces the availability of AA for eicosanoid production.*

In plain English, what this means is that the more Omega-3 fat you eat, the less Omega-6 will be available to the tissues to produce inflammation. Omega-6 is pro-inflammatory, while Omega-3 is neutral. A diet with a lot of Omega-6 and not much Omega-3 will increase inflammation. A diet of a lot of Omega-3 and not much Omega-6 will reduce inflammation.

Segment 2: More causes of inflammation and what you can do about it. Previously we talked about what inflammation is and some of the major causes. You will recall that inflammation is a normal healing response of the immune system, the beginning of a cascade of reactions to bring thousands of troops to the site of the problem, fight the good fight, then return home and get ready for the next call to action. If they stay on site, abnormal tissue damage occurs and overwhelms the body's healing capabilities. Chronic inflammation could be the cause of almost every lifestyle issue we face. Now we will continue with more potential causes and what you can do to help control levels of inflammation in the body.

Trans Fats, or man-made fats, disrupt biological function at the cellular level, causing cell death which can lead to inflammation due to immune system disruption.

Fast Carbs. A fast carb is a carbohydrate that quickly converts into sugar (glucose) in your blood stream. Of course, if you eat or drink sugar, that is a really fast carb. Processed white flour from wheat is a really fast carb, almost like sugar. White rice is a fast carb. White russet baked potatoes are not as fast as grains but still up there. Boiled or steamed sweet potatoes are not fast carbs, one because they are not baked, as baking changes the chemical structure of the sugar molecules in the potatoes, and two, there is less starch in them and three, because of all the other nutrients in the sweet potato slows the absorption of sugars into your blood stream. But anyways, fast carbs spikes your blood glucose levels which spikes your insulin levels which increases inflammatory messengers in your body.

Dietary Arachidonic Acid (AA). AA is one of the Omega 6s. And as you have learned from above, too much Omega 6s are bad for you, especially this one. AA is prevalent in farm raised fish and commercial beef feeding practices, so eat only wild caught fish, especially salmon, which is high in Omega 3s and grass-fed beef. You can Google foods high in AA for more suggestions on how to reduce intake of AA in your diet.

Leaky Gut. A leaky gut is one where gaps appear in the damaged lining of your intestinal track. That damage can be caused by a number of factors: toxins in your foods/drinks, bacterial infections, pesticides (especially glyphosate from GMOs), lack of probiotics, poor hydrochloric acid production or enzyme production in your stomach and digestive system, autoimmune conditions such as IBD and Crohn's Disease and others. It takes a specialist to help you figure out exactly what the cause and remedy is. And, the end result is undigested food proteins getting into your blood stream and lymph, that your immune system sees as foreign invaders and calls in the troops, setting off an inflammatory reaction. So, if you do not fix the leaky gut, you now have chronic inflammation.

Human Fat Cells. As mentioned before, we are learning now that our body fat cells have organ like functions especially white fat cells, not brown fat cells (see item below). They secrete substances into our blood stream, including hormones, making them endocrine organs. Some of those substances are pro inflammatory.

Homocysteine. This is a bit complicated but worth understanding at a basic level. Dr. Ben Kim describes it this way: Homocysteine is an amino acid that your body makes from another amino acid called methionine. You obtain methionine from many of the protein-dense foods that you eat on a regular basis, such as sunflower seeds, eggs, and fish. When your body does not efficiently convert homocysteine into SAMe and glutathione, the amount of homocysteine in your blood rises.

1) **High Homocysteine Speeds Up Oxidation and Aging**

Normal metabolic processes that occur in your body are constantly producing free radicals, which are unstable forms of oxygen, also called oxidants. The pace at which you age depends in large part on your body's ability to protect its tissues against these free radicals. High homocysteine significantly increases free-radical oxidation in your body and the damage that comes with it.

2) **High Homocysteine Causes Damage to Your Arteries**

High blood levels of homocysteine can damage cholesterol that is found in your blood, which can lead to direct damage of the walls of your arteries. This can lead to a series of reactions that results in thickening of the walls of your arteries, leaving less room for proper circulation. This whole process is commonly referred to as atherosclerosis.

High homocysteine can also cause your blood to have a higher than normal tendency to clot, which increases your risk of developing a dangerous clot that could lead to a stroke.

Finally, high homocysteine is known to significantly lower nitric oxide in your blood. Nitric oxide is a gas that is critical to maintaining healthy and flexible arterial walls.

3) **High Homocysteine Causes Your Immune System to Weaken**

When a high blood level of homocysteine is the result of inefficient conversion of homocysteine to glutathione, your body has less glutathione and the antioxidant activity that it provides. With less glutathione and antioxidant activity in your blood, your cells are more susceptible to damage by free radicals, which accelerates overall aging.

4) **High Homocysteine Increases Pain and Inflammation**

A high blood level of homocysteine promotes higher blood levels of arachidonic acid and prostaglandin E_2 (PGE_2), which are chemicals that your body uses to promote inflammation. While inflammation is necessary for healing in the short term, chronic inflammation can cause lasting structural damage to various tissues like your arteries, joints, and nerves.

Excessive Fibrin. When you are injured or have surgery, the body uses fibrin to help it heal. This is normal and healthy, but with poor blood flow and depleted enzyme activity the fibrin starts to accumulate. This excess fibrin causes a physical restriction of blood flow. The red blood cells get caught in this web and ultimately cannot get into the capillaries to oxygenate and nourish your muscles and **remove the metabolic waste. It is this metabolic waste** that causes inflammation and pain, leading to a chronic inflammatory condition.

Weight Loss: We are discovering that one of the many obstacles to weight loss is the inability to convert white fat into brown fat. Brown fat contains way more iron loaded mitochondria than white fat (that is what makes them brown), making it possible to burn off that brown fat quickly. Things to increase brown fat are: exercising, which can convert white-yellow fat to a more metabolically active brown fat; getting enough high-quality sleep, as proper melatonin production influences the production of brown fat; and exposing yourself to the cold regularly, such as exercising outdoors in the wintertime or in a cold room. Lowering the temperature in your living and working spaces is another tip. Turning your shower to colder water at the end of a shower (start running the cold water over your legs first, then move to other parts).

And they now understand that inflammation can hold up that conversion from white fat to brown fat. So, getting your inflammation down may be your best bet for that stubborn weight that just will not go away, especially if you eat a reasonable amount of calories and exercise regularly and your thyroid is in good health.

So briefly, here are some things you can do to lower your inflammation:

- Increase your Omega 3s through plant based and fish-based foods. Flax oil, flax seeds, certain algae and chia seeds are high in plant-based Omega 3, plus high in fiber, an extra bonus. Wild salmon, sardines, anchovies, fish oil, krill oil are high in animal Omega 3s.

- Lower your Omega 6s. See chart above plus google "foods high in AA".
- Turmeric/curcumin are extremely anti-inflammatory. Add them to your food directly or take them as supplements.
- GLA is an Omega 6, but when taken with Omega 3s, it is anti-inflammatory. You can get it from borage oil.

Meditate for few minutes two or three times a day. Try deep breathing 5 times in a row, counting to 5 each breath in, hold for 5, then release for a count of 5. Do this several times a day.

Eliminate GMOs and eat organic as much as possible. Drink filtered water.

Go to bed early, get more sleep than you think you need for survival. Plan a time on your weekend to do nothing but rest and relax, listen to music or visit with friends, go for a walk, dance, or whatever is relaxing to you.

Exercise. Moderate amounts of exercise are highly anti-inflammatory. Only 20 minutes a day can really help modulate chronic inflammation.

Lower excess fat in your body. Contact me if you want suggestions on how to do that.

Get your gut health in order. If you have burning, reflux, excessive gas, burping, bloating, irritation, constipation, loose stools, or pain in that area, try and get it resolved. There are many strategies to help you get back to good intestinal health.

Keep homocysteine levels in check by some of the above plus: Being sure to have reliable whole food sources or supplements of the following nutrients in your diet:

- Folate
- Vitamin B12
- Vitamin B6

- Vitamin B2
- Zinc
- Magnesium
- TMG (trimethylglycine - from choline)

Keep your digestive and systemic enzymes at a good level by eating lots of raw food and/or taking an enzyme supplement.

Eliminate chronic infections (including gum disease), heavy metals and parasites from your system.

To see how you are doing, check your Blood CRP levels and Homocysteine levels on your next physical. You are looking for numbers below 1 for CRP and below 9 for Homocysteine levels.

CHAPTER 9

The Multiple Causes of Fatigue

This is a tough topic because so many factors can cause this issue, so hold on to your green smoothie for a firehose of information. I do my best to synthesize into understandable themes. This theme and message is: do not accept feeling off or bad as a normal part of living, or aging, or life in America, life in the big city, life with long commuting, life with a particular job or whatever. It is not. It is a sign your body is giving you that something needs to be fixed, that a change is required, that whatever you are doing is not working.

These problems can persist for years at the same level, can get worse over time or quickly progress to much more serious illness, so it is best to pay attention to these signals and get them fixed. Acid reflux is not normal, gas and bloating are not normal, constipation/diarrhea is not normal, pain in your joints, nerve pain, long term muscle pain, abdominal discomfort, severe allergies, minor but persistent injuries; constant headaches… all of these are not normal. But, for now, I am talking about brain fog, unclear thinking, memory issues, low energy levels and cravings. These are not normal.

There are many possible reasons you may be experiencing these symptoms and with persistence and effort, you can improve and hopefully regain optimum performance; even if you have early onset Alzheimer's. We know now, this is treatable, especially if it is in one of two categories.

There are many people over 80 who have no brain fog and good energy levels, so we know it is possible to keep your brain healthy in your later years. Don't let the Norm Syndrome keep you from feeling better. So, let's get down to it, buckle your seat belt and see what could be causing your loss of function.

Here are four of the top offenders: Inflammation (see my earlier chapter on this), mitochondrial performance (our energy factory), gut health (all disease begins here) and age ((mitochondrial function goes down as we age, and inflammation follows due to increased oxidants (like Reactive Oxygen Species) being released.)) Since brain and heart and eyes have some of the highest density of mitochondria in the body…then leaking of electrons (oxidants) are highest there as we get over 40. So naturally these are the areas that are going to suffer the most from poor performing energy factories. Your job is to find your kryptonite (a Dave Asprey term) that affects this.

I thank Dave Asprey and Dr. Mark Atkinson for much of this information but have added in data from many other sources. What could be affecting inflammation, mitochondrial performance and gut health and even accelerated aging? Here are things to look for:

First, look to environmental causes such as air pollution, mold, water quality and environmental toxins. Mold alone can bring you to your knees. If your house has ever been flooded, or you work in an old broken-down work space, you may need to test it for mold. Your genes may make you especially sensitive whereas the person next to you is perfectly fine. You may need a drastic change to get away from it. If you find yourself feeling remarkably better sleeping in a different location or leaving your workspace, think mold. There are air purifiers now that kill mold.

And there are effective mold killing sprays that are non-toxic that you can spray throughout your house. But if the mold is coming from behind your walls, you will have to have your drywall replaced (expensive but necessary).

Coffee and peanut butter can be sources of mold, plus old food left the fridge too long. There are mold free coffee beans now on the market. Eliminate as many toxic/manmade compounds from your house and food as possible.

Of course, there is always the possibility of sensitivity to foods as well with gluten, dairy, refined sugar, lectins (proteins from certain plants that bind to refined carbs). Many of these sensitivities are genetic. Lectins can directly influence mitochondrial health if you are sensitive to them. What are you eating 24 to 48 hours before brain fog? Keep a journal if you have to and see if you can't track down the offending foods. You may need to try an elimination diet, eliminating most categories of food and starting with the most basic and easy to eat food for a few weeks and then adding on one at a time to see what is bugging you.

Believe me, there is an optimum diet and nutrition plan out there that will make you sing, you will want to find it. Be your own doctor, experiment with different combinations. Once you find it, keep it out of your diet until you can heal your gut. Then you can re-enter it into your diet slowly and see how you feel. Let your body be your guide.

Or, you could have nutritional deficiencies. Try taking large amounts of a multivitamin/mineral product and see if that helps, then you can slow down your dose if you see that it is helping.

Exercise. Are you moving, taking the stairs, taking a walk, getting circulation, riding a bike, doing yoga, rebounding/using a vibrating plate? Exercise can make a huge difference in brain function. Getting your blood moving creates shear forces in your arteries, causing them to release compounds that help the brain grow and lower inflammation.

It can also be a tremendous breakthrough for depression. Even if you don't (and you won't!) feel like exercising if you are depressed, force yourself. You may be amazed at the results. Do whatever your body allows you to do. I have tons of injuries and yet still manage to find ways to work around them to get my blood circulating. Moving and strength building causes mitochondrial density to grow, adding energy to your system, increasing testosterone (if you don't overdo it) bringing more oxygen to your tissues and burn fat passively when you are sitting around. Go for a walk in the sun. Lift heavier stuff twice a week for 10 to 15 minutes a session but do so while building your core so that you end up with a balanced body. Do not injure yourself, a little bit at a time.

What about lighting? Are LED's bothering you? Blue light late at night and new bright LEDs in TV and computer screens can be too much for your eyes and that energy feeds into your brain. You need your rest and you need to prepare your body for sleep. Consider the color of the sun as it sets, it's red right? Not blue. Red is preparing your nervous system for rest and regeneration so you can take full advantage of your night repair cycle. You need complete darkness when you sleep, no blinking or lit LEDs, no light from street lights coming in through your eyelids. Wear eye shades or blue light blockers after the sun sets if you must to help prepare your body for rest, sleep and regeneration.

Brain function can benefit from more ketones. Ketones are a by-product of metabolizing Medium Chain Triglycerides, found in coconut oil or you can buy ketones directly as "exogenous ketones." But they are expensive if you buy ketones directly. Or, look into nootropics (like aniracetam) and smart drugs. If you feel tired, can't find the right word, get moody, forget things easily, distract easily…that's not good. Some feel that is normal, thinking nothing of it. It is our own ability to deceive ourselves, because we are not in the hospital, so we must be OK. People get used to pain and think that is normal. Do not be normal. You want to feel good, be clear headed, have energy. If that is not normal, then you want to be abnormal.

Medications or combinations of them can cause brain fog, energy problems. Look at side effects of meds. Alcohol and illicit drugs can also cause this.

Candida, small intestinal bacteria overgrowth, dental, gut and blood infections, gingivitis, all can cause brain fog. Try a week of natural antibiotics like colloidal silver, or oil pulling for your gums if they are soar. Sore gums are not normal. Cracked teeth are not normal. Do not underestimate the destructive effects of oral health. Heavy metals coming from your teeth or bacteria-infected gums and teeth can eventually kill you.

Start with eliminating stuff that makes you weak. Then add in efforts that increase efficiency and strengthening of mitochondrial function, like removing sugar, eliminating all processed oils and adding good fats. Get enough polyphenols from bright-colored veggies, berries and coffee (use decaf if the caffeine bothers you). Even decaf has good sources of polyphenols, but don't use milk because it sticks to polyphenols. As I have said before, look for coffee brands that are free of mold. Have a big plate of veggies with some good fat, like avocado, cold flax oil, organic olive oil or coconut oil to increase your absorption of polyphenols.

Stress can cause problems; do things to relax, have fun, spend time with friends, commune with nature, focus on your breath to quiet your mind, dance, any number of things to take a break for a while from a normally chaotic mental environment.

Your energy/brain fog could be coming from a hormonal imbalance. DHEA, testosterone, thyroid (drives energy production in the body), progesterone, estrogen. Go in for a hormonal work-up and see how you are doing. Family or emotional stress can stop mitochondria from doing the repair cycle and can really slow you down over time. Excess cortisol from constant stress can exhaust your adrenals or something in your hypothalamus/pituitary/adrenal system, leaving you at times with zero energy levels. Don't let that happen, it is hell to recover from.

Anxiety/Depression

PTSD after a dramatic event? It may feel normal to you, may have been present from childhood. Thyroid, medications? Hypoglycemic? Need to work on this. Try passion flower, lemon balm, magnesium, Box Breathing (I can teach you how.), L-theanine.

Personality disorders? Take care of them, perhaps with cognitive behavioral therapy. You can check out books on this subject. Many are self-help. Spend more time in your healing mode (parasympathetic instead of sympathetic).

EMDR, HRV training from Heart Math called Inner Balance. Brain spotting, neuro feeback techniques. Holosync, tapping can help get you into a relaxed state. Take your attention off the story and locate where the stress or tension is in your body and say to it, "I am pleased you are here," then you get a sense of where that tension wants to exit, then it will start moving and pour out of you, usually out your mouth. Neurogenic tremoring or shaking can help. Check it out on the internet. Natural tremoring can discharge negative energy and return to a calmer state. Start with one or two things first, chart your progress and notice how you start in the right direction. Exercise can help dump adrenal stress (stress caused by hormones from adrenals.).

According to Tara Thorne, a registered holistic nutritionist, common herbs can really help with depression/anxiety:

turmeric/curcumin; rosemary. It's not only consuming rosemary that produces the mental health benefits: rosemary essential oil has also proven powerful in reducing stress and anxiety. This was reflected in a study involving graduate nursing students who, after being exposed to rosemary essential oil, scored lower on anxiety tests as well as personal anxiety statements and also exhibited reduced pulse rates. Another study, which used rosemary extract in combination with lavender, marjoram, eucalyptus, and peppermint, showed significant decreases in depression scores in the group of people exposed to the essential oil combination; and saffron.

Also, in one study of 470 elderly men, those who ate about 2.3 grams of cocoa powder per day over five years had significantly lower blood pressure translating to a 45-50% decrease in cardiovascular and all-cause risk.

The authors attribute the vasodilation effects of chocolate to an increase in nitric oxide induced by the cacao flavanols.

The researchers also tested a combination of 60% cacao chocolate and 128 mg of L-theanine, an amino acid found in green tea. Studies show L-theanine produces calming alpha waves in the brain and reduces blood pressure.

Further, according to Dr. Mercola:

- Vitamin D can improve a number of brain disorders, including depression and Alzheimer's disease.
- Seniors with severe vitamin D deficiency may raise their risk for dementia by 125 percent.
- Low vitamin D levels also predispose you to depression.
- An eight-year-long study shows that higher levels of depression translate into greater risk for dementia later on.

- Having a vitamin D level below 20 ng/mL may raise your risk for depression by 85 percent, compared to having a vitamin D level greater than 30 ng/mL.
- Vitamin D supplementation has been found to reduce both depression and diabetic pain. It can also help prevent the progression of prediabetes into full blown diabetes.

One more quick culprit that hits thousands if not millions that I kind of skimmed over and cannot ignore is heavy metals. It is a deep and complicated topic. Keep in mind our exposure to heavy metals increases every year and there are many sources. It is well worth your effort to get tested in a hair analysis and challenge urine analysis (where a chelator is ingested and pulls heavy metals into your urine for analysis and detection). Once detected, there are many ways to get them out of your system, from dental procedures to infrared saunas to zeolite to IV chelators and other compounds known for heavy metal removals. Or, you can be like me, assume you have constant exposure and start a program of heavy metal removal on some regular schedule. Maybe I will devote an entire chapter on this topic in a later version. Let me know if that is of interest.

So, don't be normal and accept your discomfort. Start working on it piece by piece, be it emotional discomfort or physical or brain disorders. Do your research and/or work with a professional to get your issues resolved.

CHAPTER 10

Overcoming Candida

As you may know, both friendly and unhealthy micro-organisms exist in your body in a delicate balance giving you life and sustenance while helping to maintain and train your immune system. In fact, these organisms way outnumber your own human cells 10 to one. In terms of genetics, their DNA outnumber ours 100 to one. That is incredible! We also know there is a constant exchange of DNA between us and them, making us an intricate link in the micro/plant/animal kingdom. There is no escaping it.

This has caused me to revise my belief in Darwin's conclusion of survival of the fittest. Now, I think evolution is survival due to a cooperative/sharing arrangement between everything alive at the genetic level. Thanks to the constant sharing of genetic material facilitated by micro-organisms as the communication bus, needed improvements are transferred to our own genetics, helping us adjust to changing environments. But I diverge.

Many factors weaken our immunity and upset this balance...the chemicals we add to our food and environment, fast-food diets, the stress in our daily lives, and the widespread use of medicines, especially antibiotics and hormones. When the body is in this weakened state, the unfriendly bacteria or fungus can multiply quickly, producing symptoms such as headaches, nausea, skin rashes, and food allergies, fatigue, mood disorders, depression as well as other potentially more serious disorders.

Most of us begin life with a clean bill of health with plentiful healthy bacteria in our initial inoculation, the birth canal, which perhaps contains bacteria from millions of years ago. Think about it, besides inheriting genetics and epigenetics (see next chapter) from all previous generations, you also inherit bacteria from the beginning of human reproduction; through intercourse, you not only inherit your mom's vaginal bacteria, but your dad's as well. Your mother's milk promotes healthy bacteria and subdues unhealthy bacteria. As it continues, the healthy bacteria gain a foothold in the baby's digestive tract and in the vagina of the females.

It takes about three months for an inner ecosystem to settle in, and after this period of time, the microbiome starts to resemble the mothers. This points to the importance of the mother having the best possible health prior to and during pregnancy. The baby's beneficial bacteria thrive on natural sugars from breast milk and then from food. These sugars along with soluble fiber feed the good bacteria, which in turn provide us with many good things like B vitamins and short chain fatty acids such as Acetate and Lactate which are used as fuel. Another is Propionate which travels to the liver and helps regulate cholesterol. Butyrate helps regulate energy, cholesterol and hormone production, and programmed cell death to prevent colon cancer.

As we grow older, the balance evolves and changes as it should, and our diets have direct and immediate influence over the species of bacteria in our gut. Some things change the balance in unfavorable ways. Long term antibiotics give rise to the invasion of new species or allow normally healthy low levels of bad bacteria and microbes to flourish into unhealthy levels, invading your system and secreting toxins that cause havoc in your system and giving rise to symptoms. Candida is one of these micro-organisms; a yeast or fungus that feeds on and thrives on sugar.

Candida, a single cell organism, reproduces asexually and thrives on some of the body's by-products: dead tissue and sugars from food. Unless its source of food is eliminated, it quickly monopolizes entire bodily systems, and can cause mild to severe discomfort. If it really gets out of control, it is frequently a major cause of death, especially in victims of cancer and AIDS. But it can also hijack your immune system, causing it to be distracted, focusing too much on fighting Candida and leaving you open to other infections and cancer.

In her book, *The Body Ecology Diet*, Donna Gates lists 7 principles of eating and healing to recover from this terrible affliction of an epidemic of microbiome imbalances and more specifically Candida run-away trains.

1. **Expansion and Contraction:** Certain foods such as salt, meat and poultry, cause the body to contract or tighten. When the body is too tight, circulation slows and elimination of waste comes to a standstill (constipation). Other foods like sugar, alcohol and coffee, cause the body to expand and relax. People who eat large amounts of contracting foods, develop craving for expansion foods. What we need, is to stay in balance. (See by 16th Law of Life.)

2. **Acid/Alkaline:** This is a deep topic that deserves an entire chapter, so let me just say that being overly acidic causes all sorts of problems in the body, as each part of your body requires different pH levels, including healthy bacteria.

3. **Uniqueness:** Everyone is different, so you need to find the diet that works best for you.

4. **Cleansing:** The Body Ecology Diet encourages you to welcome cleansings, because they always result in a higher level of health and immunity.

5. **Proper Food Combining**: Certain combinations of food result in cleaner digesting, less fermentation of foods in the digestive tract and therefore less food for Candida, keeping it in check. The main one I live by is never eat animal protein with starchy vegetables and grains and what is the mainstay of western life? Meat and potatoes. No wonder we have issues!!

6. **The 80/20 Principle**: Eat until your stomach is 80 percent full, leaving 20% for digesting. Also, 80% of the food on your plate should be vegetables, 20% proteins/grains/ starchy vegetables.

7. **Take It Step by Step:** The first steps are to create a hearty inner ecosystem in your intestines, create energy by nourishing your adrenals and thyroid, conquer infections… especially fungal infections, and cleanse.

One of the great missing links in all other systems of health is that of fermented foods. It is a great source of probiotics and you can't get too much of it. It is also a great way to get rid of acid reflux and heal ulcers, re-establishing the right balance of bacteria in your stomach and intestinal tract.

If you have tried many things and have not gotten better, or you just want to improve your health to the next level, I highly recommend picking up a copy of *The Body Ecology Diet* from Donna Gates.

CHAPTER 11

Epigenetics Part 1

You Have Control Over Your Genetic Expression

In this chapter, we are delving into the cell, into the world of DNA and control of our health through genetic expression. And yes, as science is learning, we do have a huge influence over genetic expression, both positive and negative. This whole emerging field called Epigenetics is giving us tremendous insights into why our children are becoming increasingly sicker and how one can tailor health care to each individual (called nutrigenomics (nutrition based on someone's genes)) and pharmacogenomics (drug therapy based on someone's genes)).

Epigenetics is the study of potentially inheritable changes in gene expression (in other words, some genes are active or "turned on" versus inactive genes or "turned off") that does not involve changes to the underlying DNA genetic code — or in other words, a change in phenotype (which genes are read and therefore expressed) without a change in genotype (the order of the DNA code). Think in terms of the DNA being our hardware and epigenetic markers as being our software.

What we are talking about are markers that attach to genes causing them to unwind and be read or to close up and be hidden. Epigenetic change is a regular and natural occurrence essential to good health and cell identity but can be influenced by several factors including age, the lifestyle, dietary intake, drug therapies we are on, environmental toxins, even our beliefs/emotions and disease state.

To help understand the importance of genetic markers, you need to understand that epigenetic modifications can come in two flavors; either tell stem cells(originating cells that do not yet have an assignment for what function to fulfill in the body) what to become (for example end up as skin cells, liver cells, brain cells, nerve cells). Or, epigenetic change can have damaging effects that can result in diseases like cancer or accelerated aging.

Each one of our cells in our body has the same exact hardware code in our DNA, exactly the same in every cell. What tells them you are a liver cell and you are an eye cell? It is the markers/tags that attach to the DNA that controls what is read and what is hidden, that gives our cells a specific identity. There are at least three systems currently considered to initiate and sustain epigenetic change: 1) DNA methylation, 2) histone modification and 3) non-coding RNA (ncRNA).

We are going to go over each of these because our health depends on the correct set of markers or tags being present at any given time. Now please understand, science is not at the point of understanding this software well enough to adjust singular tags to affect a particular result. But we do know many of the right nutrients to include in our diet that are the building blocks for these tags, allowing the body to design and implement the best software for every condition.

New and ongoing research is continuously uncovering the role of epigenetics in a variety of human disorders and fatal diseases. But before we launch into what each of these three types of influences actually are and how we can supply the building blocks to help the body have healthy genetic expression versus disease causing expression, we probably first need to review the basics about DNA and genes and protein manufacture and how that all works so you can understand epigenetic influences on those genes.

So, as a quick review (or maybe your first exposure), your DNA mainly is composed of a sequence of compounds called bases. There are four of them. And the order of those bases determines which proteins are produced by any given gene. The gene is nothing more than a segment of DNA that is composed of any number of bases that are needed to produce a particular protein. The DNA from one human cell, if extended would cover about six feet in length, so to compact it all into the cell nucleus (a very, very tight space), we use a spooling technology, winding the DNA around a body called a histone.

In fact, there are many histones in the nucleus, each winding several segments of thread (the DNA) around each spool (the histone). When the cell is ready to make another protein, the DNA unwinds at the right place, the base sequence is read and then translated into an exact sequence of amino acids that chain together to make exactly the right protein (our proteins are nothing more than a sequence of amino acids dictated by the DNA). And as you may know, proteins are the building blocks of life, supplying everything from muscles, connective tissue, to a glue that holds tissue together, to immune system components, to scaffolding for cell structure, to channels in cell membranes allowing nutrients to pass in and out of cells, to sensors sitting on top of your cells, to messengers inside your cells relaying information coming in from outside the cell, and to enzymes that digest our food and other metabolic enzymes that keep chemical reactions humming in our entire body.

All these different proteins are coded for by some segment of our DNA, due to the order of the four bases. Pretty hard to believe that just four different bases could code for so many different proteins, but when you group the four bases together in the thousands in different sequences along the DNA double helix, you can begin to see the number of combinations that are possible.

But when we are talking about Epigenetics, we are talking about markers on these genes or Histones that cause them to wind up tightly on the spools and hide DNA from translation, or open DNA for reading and protein production. Do not get this confused with the ability to discover what your DNA code is and possible abnormal sequencing of the bases. This is what seems to be the rage now, getting your DNA analyzed for ancestry or detection of abnormal genes or base sequencing, determining your hardware, which is an entirely different discussion but related to epigenetics, your software.

Why is it related? Because an abnormal gene could lower your ability to produce genetic markers that control gene expression. For example, if you have an abnormal gene that lowers your ability to produce a protein enzyme (all enzymes are proteins) called MTHFR, you will have what is called a methylation issue which will result in a lowered amount of Methyl groups (one carbon, 3 hydrogens (CH3)) in your body. Methyl groups are key epigenetic markers that tend to hide or tighten DNA strands around the spools, preventing them from being translated.

On the other hand, if you have a genetic defect that causes a decrease in the production of a different marker called an acetyl group, then you will be less able to open a gene for translation. So, knowing that your genetics are abnormal and therefore not producing enough methyl groups for example, is there anything you can do in the nutrition world to compensate for this? Yes, absolutely. That is nutrigenomics or adding the right nutrients to your diet to supply your body the missing compounds that get around the lack of production due to a hardware defect. Or perhaps drugs can be designed to bypass this or that process to crank up methyl production, that is pharmacogenomics.

Also, we are learning that gene coding can also make you more sensitive to certain drugs because you cannot metabolize certain drugs as well as other people. Doctors are now using this information for proper drug dosing tailored to each individual. We are only at the very tip of the iceberg in understanding all this and how to use this knowledge to tweak our nutritional/drug protocols to get the most out of our hardware and supply the right building blocks, so our bodies can adjust the software as needed.

And we now know that this software is inheritable at least to the fourth generation and probably more. And that the damage from bad software is cumulative if it is not fixed, getting worse in each generation. We are either born at a disadvantage, carrying the negative markers of our nutritionally and psychologically starved ancestors (emotional trauma changes epigenetic markers) from several generations, or we are blessed with healthy ancestors whose software was in excellent condition at the time of conception. Markers are passed from both the father and mother, so if we want to help our offspring have the best start in life, we need the healthiest lifestyles prior to conception.

This could explain why our kids for the first time in recorded medical history, are not supposed to exceed our average age. They are getting sicker younger, many of them having trouble conceiving and bearing children of their own, exactly what a researcher found in the 1940s in a famous study called Pottinger's cats, although at that time, we did not know why.

The experiment included 900 cats over four generations and was well documented by Dr. Pottenger. The cats were divided into five groups. All the groups were supplied the same basic minimal diet, but the major portion of the diets were varied. Two of the groups were fed whole foods (raw milk and meat – real foods for cats). The other three groups were given processed foods: pasteurized, evaporated and condensed milk.

All four generations of the raw meat and raw milk groups remained healthy throughout their normal lifespans. The first generation of all three processed food groups developed diseases and illnesses near the end of their lives. The second generation of all three processed food groups developed diseases and illnesses in the middle of their lives. The third generation of all three processed food groups developed diseases and illnesses in the beginning of their lives and many died before six months of age.

There was no fourth generation in any of the three processed food groups. Either the third-generation parents were sterile, or the fourth-generation cats died before birth! Remember, all four generations of the raw food groups were healthy throughout their normal lifespans.

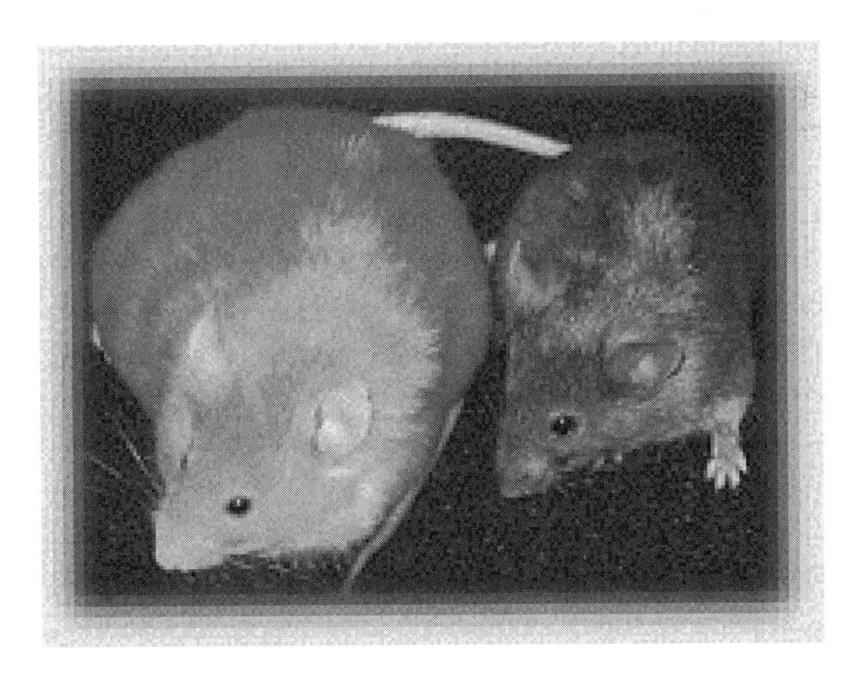

We also see dramatic changes in epigenetic influence of the agouti gene in mice. For instance, in normal, healthy lean brown mice, the agouti genes are kept in the "off" position by the epigenome, which attaches methyl groups to the corresponding regions of DNA, resulting in the DNA's compaction to prevent transcription. In yellow and/or obese mice, however, the same exact genes are not methylated; thus, these genes are expressed or "turned on." The turning on of this single gene results in an apparent freak of nature.

Mice whose agouti gene is "on" are also more likely to suffer from diabetes and cancer as adults. Having an adequate supply of methyl groups makes a dramatic difference in these genetically identical mice. Kind of makes me wonder what our hidden potential is as humans, if we had perfect gene expression.

Another example is from the bees. The only difference between the Queen Bee and the workers is Royal Jelly. That is it. They are genetically identical. That is what nutrition can do for the expression of genes.

To sum up, we know our epigenetic software is inheritable and has a huge influence on our health and hundreds of other parameters with dramatic swings possible in gene expression. Next chapter, we will go into each of those three factors that make up our epigenetic software and what are some of the emerging nutritional/lifestyle factors that we can do to optimize our genetic expression. We already talked about two of the markers, methyl groups which tend to hide genes and acetyl groups which tend to expose genes. What do we need to be doing to give our body the best chance in design of the best software? One is prevention and two is supplementation...great subjects for Epigenetics Part 2.

CHAPTER 12

EPIGENETICS PART 2

A More Complete Understanding

This is complicated stuff!! Do not feel bad if it takes a while to digest it. In Epigenetics Part 1, we delved deep into cellular function and how the DNA is translated into proteins. We talked about how cell identity is determined by your software tags that determine which DNA is exposed and which DNA is hidden and how that not only gives the stem cell its mission in life (kidney, nerve, heart etc.) but also has a dramatic effect over your overall health. I showed that these effects are cumulative and inheritable over the generations. I talked about two of the three genetic markers or tags, the methyl groups which tend to close down or hide DNA and acetyl groups which tend to expose or open up DNA for translation into proteins.

Let's continue. Since you inherit your markers from your parents, and you create your markers yourself throughout your life starting in the womb at conception, science today really does not know which tag comes from which source. They really have at least three generations of information to sort out at any given time in the child or embryo; tags from mom and dad, tags from grandparents and tags from food/conditions/fluids during embryonic development. But they do have some evidence to go by. For example, obese men have different markers than slender men and we know now that they pass on these markers to their offspring.

In Part 1, I told you about the three categories of epigenetic influence, the DNA tags, the Histone Tags and the non-coding RNA influence. The DNA tags that lock on to a particular base in your DNA are the Methyl Groups, the Histone tags are the Acetyl Groups. Let's talk briefly about the third category of genetic expression, non-coding RNA. If you remember, RNA reads the base sequence in your hardware and then translates that into a protein. So, a non-coding RNA reads a DNA base sequence and does not produce a protein. What I am really saying is that there are large segments of your DNA that are Dark Matter, that perform jobs other than protein production and frankly, we are just beginning to understand what those jobs are, one of which is to control software tags. Surprisingly, about 98.5% of the genome does not code for proteins!!

One kind of non-coding RNA is known as microRNA and is believed capable of acting as a master regulator of gene expression across the plant and animal kingdoms. I find it pretty amazing that only about 1.5% of our entire DNA is actually used to produce proteins. What is the rest doing? There are not even enough protein coding genes (about 20,000) to account for some 100,000 proteins found in the human body. We are like a baby in the woods when comes to understanding our genetic code. All of this has been revealed as a result of the miracle of now being able to quickly analyze a human's entire genome.

Our dark matter in our genes is kind of like the dark matter in the universe, almost a complete mystery to us. As the great researcher and biological philosopher Sayer Ji has said, "And why would this be so, if not for a purpose? Life does not concern itself with producing anything without reason.

A new paper suggests this as a possible answer:

The function of these non-coding RNAs is largely unknown. Can it be hypothesized that a function of the non- coding ("dark matter") would be the mediation of inter-individual, inter-species or cross-kingdom communication? Not only that, microRNAs (non-coding) can travel between cell types within the body (soma to germline), but (also) between species.

As microRNAs are major products of the non-protein coding part of the genome, these could be the primary mediators of epigenetic information traversing tissues, different individuals and even species, and thus linking different organisms. It cannot be excluded that beside microRNAs, other non-coding RNA molecules (e.g. long non-coding RNA molecules instead of micro RNA) might also be involved in mediating genomic information, but small molecular weight microRNAs would be the most suitable for such communication given their stability. "

These are your three currently known epigenetic influences. The field of epigenetics is quickly growing and with it the understanding that both the environment, drugs and individual lifestyle can also directly interact with the genome to influence epigenetic change. For example, in some people, *Scientific American* in May 2017, reported that aspirin investigators have identified about 60 genes that are turned on or off in response to taking aspirin. There is so much we don't know.

In general, genetic expression changes may be reflected at various stages throughout a person's life and even in later generations. For example, human epidemiological studies have provided evidence that prenatal and early postnatal environmental factors influence the adult risk of developing various chronic diseases and behavioral disorders. Studies have shown that children born during the period of the Dutch famine from 1944-

1945 have increased rates of coronary heart disease and obesity after maternal exposure to famine during early pregnancy compared to those not exposed to famine.

Less DNA methylation of the insulin-like growth factor II (IGF2) gene, a well-characterized epigenetic locus, was found to be associated with this exposure. Likewise, adults that were prenatally exposed to famine conditions have also been reported to have significantly higher incidence of schizophrenia.

Clinical Applications – Some Epigenetic Diseases

Cancer. Cancer was the first human disease to be linked to epigenetics. Studies performed by Feinberg and Vogelstein in 1983, using primary human tumor tissues, found that genes of colorectal cancer cells were substantially hypomethylated (under) compared with normal tissues. DNA hypomethylation can activate oncogenes and initiate chromosome instability, whereas DNA hypermethylation (over) initiates silencing of tumor suppressor genes. An accumulation of genetic and epigenetic errors can transform a normal cell into an invasive or metastatic tumor cell. Additionally, DNA methylation patterns may cause abnormal expression of cancer-associated genes.

Global histone modification patterns are also found to correlate with cancers such as prostate, breast, and pancreatic cancer. Subsequently, epigenetic changes can be used as biomarkers for the molecular diagnosis of early cancer. The question that arises is: does the change in genetic expression cause the cancer or does the cancer cause a change in genetic markers. This is a topic of hot research right now. I am personally on the side of the metabolic theory of cancer, meaning that it is a change in the way that a cell uses glucose (a failure of the mitochondria to produce energy) that sets off a chain reaction that changes our epigenetics, which then causes the immortality of cancer cells.

Mental Retardation Disorders. Epigenetic changes are also linked to several disorders that result in intellectual disabilities. For example, the imprint disorders Prader-Willi syndrome and Angelman syndrome, display an abnormal phenotype (software) as a result of the absence of the paternal or maternal copy of a gene, respectively. In these imprint disorders, there is a genetic deletion in chromosome 15 in a majority of patients. The same gene on the corresponding chromosome cannot compensate for the deletion because it has been turned off by methylation, an epigenetic modification. Genetic deletions inherited from the father result in Prader-Willi syndrome, and those inherited from the mother, Angelman syndrome.

Immunity & Related Disorders. There are several pieces of evidence showing that loss of epigenetic control over complex immune processes contributes to autoimmune disease

Neuropsychiatric Disorders. Epigenetic errors also play a role in the causation of complex adult psychiatric, autistic, and neurodegenerative disorders. A role for aberrant methylation mediated by folate levels has been suggested as a factor in Alzheimer's disease; also, some preliminary evidence supports a model that incorporates both genetic and epigenetic contributions in the causation of autism.

Pediatric Syndromes. In addition to epigenetic alterations, specific mutations affecting components of the epigenetic pathway have been identified that are responsible for several syndromes: DNMT3B in ICF (immunodeficiency, centromeric instability and facial anomalies) syndrome, MECP2 in Rett syndrome, ATRX in ATR-X syndrome (a-thalassemia/mental retardation syndrome, X-linked), and DNA repeats in facioscapulohumeral muscular dystrophy.

The increased knowledge and technologies in epigenetics over the last ten years allow us to better understand the interplay between epigenetic change, gene regulation, and human diseases, and will lead to the development of new approaches for molecular diagnosis and targeted treatments across the clinical spectrum.

But no epigenetic discussion would be complete without talking about a class of enzymes called Histone Deacetyleases (HDACs)---in other words, enzymes that effect your genetic expression by removing acetyl groups from Histones. Since acetyl groups tend to hide genes, removing them exposes genes. This goes back to what I was saying earlier, that our genes code for proteins (enzymes in this case) that effect tags in our software. So what we want to do from a nutrition standpoint, is to ensure these enzymes have everything they need, to do their job throughout life, exposing genes and hiding genes as appropriate.

As it turns out, a researcher from Harvard believes he broke the code on this and started his own company marketing a product called Elysium. You can go to the website to read all the biochemistry behind it, and how the compound NAD+ is critical to beneficial epigenetic control. But there are many products on the market now that have the same ingredients (building blocks of NAD) and even oral products where you take NAD directly into your system under the tongue. My point is, yes, without testing, there are things you can do to help your software. And as time goes on, there will be more and more products on the market.

What can you do to help insure your body has the best building blocks and signals to build the best software? One is avoidance of as many toxins and drugs as you can (un-natural manmade or processed substances), working through all your emotional trauma, drinking filtered water and the other is nutritional elements that have been found to influence positive genetic expression. The primary source of this information below is from Dr. Lucia Aronica, an epigenetics researcher at Stanford.

I added a few items of clarification and additions to the list from other scientific sources:

Agent	Source	Effect
Methionine (amino acid)	Sesame Seeds, Brazil Nuts, Fish, Peppers, Spinach	Good Aid to SAM Synthesis (methyl group production)
Folate	Leafy Greens, Sunflower Seeds, Baker's Yeast, Liver	Good aid to MTHF synthesis (methyl group production)
B12	Meat, Liver, Shellfish, Milk	Critical for Methyl production
B6	Meat, whole grains, veggies, nuts	Good for MTHF synthesis
SAM–e	Supplements	Good Methyl Donor
Choline	Egg Yolk, liver, Soy, Meats	Good Methyl Donor
Betaine	Wheat, Spinach, shellfish, Sugar Beets	Good for Break Down of toxic byproducts of SAM generation
Resveratrol	Wine/Red Grapes	Life preserving signaling to epigenetic tagging
Genistein	Non-GMO Soy	Removes incorrect Acetyl groups
Sulphoraphane	Broccoli	Increases good Acetyl groups
Butyrate	Fiber/Intestinal Fermentation	Increases good Acetyl groups, increasing lifespan
Diallyl Sulphate	Garlic	Increased good Acetyl groups turning on anti-cancer genes
Prescription Medications	Synthetic drugs	Unknown – but does change the tagging patterns
Environmental toxins	Hundreds	Cancer and other diseases through epigenetic changes
Smoking	Cigaretts etc.	Cancer through epigenetic changes
Betahydroxybuterate	Ketones (MCT fats/coconut oil)	Signals healthy gene expression
NAD+	Supplements (Nicotinamide Riboside)	Raises NAD+ levels, Signals healthy gene expression

Let's sum up. Your hardware can have some abnormal base sequences which can be hidden by good software. Just because you test and come up with some abnormal coding, does not mean you will come down with those associated diseases. You are made to deal with gene mutations, if your software production is in good shape.

On the other hand, some hardware coding abnormalities can actually inhibit the production of software tags, like MTHFR, which inhibits methyl group production. You can take supplements to work around these deficiencies like B complex vitamins. But in general, we need to recognize that our health depends on good software, and if we do not start out in life blessed with a great inheritance of good tags, then we need to work especially hard to control our exposure to toxins and processed foods and drugs, minimize stress and get nutrient dense foods. Extra measures, like the ones above, can help ensure the best software possible and minimize bad gene expression.

THOUGHT BREAK#4: MEDITATIONS FOR THE SOUL

Wow, that was a lot!! Let's take a break…

Breaking the bonds of stress in your life and moving into a state of positive energy is critically important for health, but easier said than done right? So here are some of my favorite meditations for you to use and ponder. Some are from a great friend and massage therapist, Elizabeth, at Touching Life, LLC in Leesburg, Virginia.

1. Immerse yourself in the flow of the universe. Let it be. —Alberto Villoldo, Ph.D.

2. Summon power and wisdom to understand the present, heal the past, and influence the course of your future.

3. Bodhisattva Prayer for Humanity"
   "May I be a guard for those who need protection
   A guide for those on the path
   A boat, a raft, a bridge for those who wish to cross the flood
   May I be a lamp in the darkness
   A resting place for the weary
   A healing medicine for all who are sick
   A vase of plenty, a tree of miracles
   And for the boundless multitudes of living beings
   May I bring sustenance and awakening
   Enduring like the earth and sky
   Until all beings are freed from sorrow
   And all are awakened."
   Now, exhale and be still for a brief moment.

4. Say out loud:
   I am a being of light.
   I am a being of love.
   I am a being of purpose.
   I am a being: here to enjoy my life and offer the best of who I am into the world.
   I am.

5. As Mother Teresa says: Give the world the best you have and it may never be enough but give it anyways, because in the final analysis, it is between you and God, it was never between you and them anyway.

6. Say, If I am doing my best to shine, it is more than enough. Visualize yourself sitting in a pyramid of life, feel the platinum ray of transmutation and peace, pouring into what your human difficulty still might be, if it is in the crown of your head, not hearing the divine, let it be healed and cleared, if it is in your third eye not able to see the world as god sees it, let's clear that, if it comes through you're not being able to speak your truth of who you are, lets clear that, if it comes from your heart where you have felt saddened and disappointed and betrayed, lets clear that, if it comes lower in the center of your power where you felt subjugated and suppressed, lets clear that; if it comes in the second chakra with your connections and your relationships, lets clear that: and if it comes from the root where you don't feel safe or connected with this beautiful earth, lets clear that. And so now in the pyramid of light, the platinum ray has allowed and offered you an opportunity for clearing. And now the chance is for each of you as you read this and the moments to follow, fill that pyramid of light with the truth of you, by saying; I AM…state your name…I AM a being of

light, I AM a being of love, I AM a being of presence and pleasure and peace and prosperity and power. And so, it is.

Let your life and this year be an incredible year of recovery, reinvention, rebuilding, regeneration and most of all Joy. You are loved. Namaste.

7. From the Lord God of my being to the Lord God of all, I now release any belief, perception, judgment or doubt, any pattern, any holding any memory, anything that no longer serves my highest good. I release you now to the healing power of the holy god. Go and be healed, be reclaimed in grace. Thank you for whatever gift you may have given to me, but I command you now to depart. And, so it is.

8. This meditation can be done anywhere and at any time. However, you may want to create a special time or a special place in your home where you will invite the Presence of God into your body, your mind and your life in a way that feels sacred to you. Feel free to tailor this meditation to fit your beliefs and your personal needs. Sit comfortably, light a candle if you wish, and breathe deeply in and out through your nose. Make sure to fill your lungs completely and to empty your lungs completely. Relax from the top of your head all the way down to the tips of your toes.

   Begin: I now invite the Presence of God into my body, my mind and my life. I ask that you fill me completely and entirely. (Take a deep breath and really feel the presence really filling and expanding you) I ask the Presence of God to take away the congestion and the darkness in my body, my mind and my life. I ask the Presence of God to clear away the congestion and the cobwebs and to leave pure light, joy and healing in every corner and place that was dark. I ask the Presence of God to open my body, to take away unnecessary tension and to heal me everywhere that healing is needed.

I ask the Presence of God to enter and to heal all my relationships and to bring strength, love and understanding to all of my relationships. I ask the Presence of God to enter and to heal my marriage and to bring strength, love and understanding to my marriage. I ask the Presence of God to fill me and to bring me lasting, joyous and supportive friendships and familial relationships. I ask the Presence of God to enter and to heal my financial situations and dealings and to fill my life with abundance so that I, in turn, may continue to give to others. I ask the Presence of God to enter and to assist me in fulfilling my soul's purpose here on earth in a joyful and harmonious manner. I invite the Presence of God to enter and fill me with energy and inspiration. I invite the Presence of God to fill me and to love through my heart, to create and serve using my hands and my body. I invite the Presence of God to speak through my voice, to hear with compassion through my ears and to see through my eyes.

Thank you for these blessings and for your comfort and support. Highest Honor and Highest Gratitude. (Now you can relax knowing that the only energy operating in your life is through the Presence of God.)

9. Our Mother Earth is available to us to help us process our negative and heavy energy in a cleansing and supportive way. We have a co-creative relationship with the earth. An example is how we give out CO_2 and receive back nourishing Oxygen. We can surrender our heavy energy to the earth and allow the earth's positively charged life force energy to fill the spaces in

our physical and energy bodies that need healing. When the weather is warm try to place a blanket down and actually lay on the earth. Lay comfortably on a blanket on the lowest level floor of your home or office if a place in nature is not available to you. Make sure to support your lower back by placing a pillow under your knees. You can also imagine that you are in your favorite place in nature if you are doing this exercise inside a building.

Take at least 10 minutes to do this exercise. Lay in a comfortable position and begin deeply and slowly filling your lungs completely and slowly emptying your lungs completely. Breathing in and out only through your nose. In your mind ask Mother Earth to take your heavy energy as you exhale and imagine the heavy energy leaving you and seeping into the ground. You can ask Mother Earth to take away what is making you ill or unhappy and anything and everything that is keeping you from living the life your soul came to this planet to enjoy and complete.

Spend a few minutes handing over everything that you need to let go. Then ask Mother Earth to begin filling you with her healing strengthening loving energy. Inhale deeply and imagine that you are drawing it up from the center of the earth and it is filling your physical and your energy bodies everywhere that you have a need for it. Spend a few minutes doing this. Now let go of heavy energy into the earth as you exhale and breathe in and fill your body with the positive earth energy as you inhale. Spend a few moments sending your love and appreciation to Mother Earth for her support and care when you feel balanced and ready to end the session.

Try to do this exercise at least once a day

10. Go to: https://www.youtube.com/watch?v=j9Mzyf_B8rQ, skip the ads and listen uninterrupted for at least 20 min if you can. Close your eyes and imagine walking out into heaven, everything you imagine heaven to be. You are surrounded by warm brighter light than you have ever known. With that light comes love, peace and joy, penetrating every fiber of your existence. You have no worries, no needs, no fears, no guilt, no anger, no frustrations… just pure blinding non-judgmental love coming through you and pouring out of you. Bask in this incredible place, bathe in its happiness, let your negative emotions run out of you, draining you of everything that has been holding you back and keeping you imprisoned in this earthly existence. Now you feel free, now your internal light is glowing, now you are melding with all that is, that ever will be. Amen…

If you have other favorite meditations, please send them in and I will try and include them in my next edition: Email me at Bob@conscioushealthclub.com.

CHAPTER 13

Natural Antibiotic and Anti-viral Protocols

We all need to learn the ancient and modern secrets to keeping our immune system healthy and fighting infection from pathogens. There are literally hundreds of scientifically proven natural compounds that act as anti-biotics and help build and keep the immune system balanced and on guard. This is especially important these days because of the anti-biotic resistant bacteria that are emerging as a world-wide health threat, killing hundreds of thousands every year (dot # 48), and the problem is getting worse all the time with the indiscriminate use of anti-biotics in our meat supply and ending up in our water supply along with overuse in general from the medical community. Experts are really worried about resistant strains.

Not only because of over use of anti-biotics, but because resistant strains can and do share their genes with other bacteria and organisms. One researcher in the 1950s dubbed it "infective heredity." Genome sequencing reveals that such horizontal transfer of DNA has been profoundly important in the history of life, and among bacteria it is especially common, with particular implications on the spread of antibiotic-resistance genes. A Japanese researcher (Watamanbe) discovered at least one mechanism for that transfer in the 1960s and called the material an "episome." This is a free-floating piece of DNA inside the cell, unattached to the chromosome. They are now called plasmids and are recognized as a major mechanism for transferal of antibiotic-resistant genes- sometimes whole packets of genes for multiple resistance- from one species of bacterium to another.

Don't get me wrong, prescription anti-biotics and anti-virals absolutely have a place in your life and can save you from terrible misery, if you really need them. For example, if you come down with the Shingles (weird dots on your skin, perhaps a rash, making your skin very painful, a very painful virus that attacks the nerves), don't mess around with it.

Go in and get some very effective antivirals to lessen the pain, shorten the duration and possibly prevent lasting damage. But over use of medical anti-biotics can ruin your health as well by wiping out vital good bacteria in your digestive tract and causing bacterial resistance. Try to overcome your typical infections or colds (which is a virus, not a bacteria) through natural means over a reasonable time frame before going to see a doc. And if you do take antibiotics, make sure follow it up quickly with a strong course of probiotics to restore your gut health.

A simple of search of GreenMedInfo will give you a list of tons of natural anti-microbial compounds, everything from high dose Vitamin C and D3, to garlic, ginger, berries, berberine, bee propolis, Manuka Honey, colloidal silver, curcumin, Allicin, Tea Tree oil, Myrr Oil, Eyucalyptis oil, Oregano oil, aloe vera, EGCG, Grape Seed Extract, Cordyceps, Beta Glucan, Clove Oil, Caprylic acid, Zinc, Cranberry juice, and Broccoli Sprout Powder, to mention a few.

I use a combination of therapies at my house when I feel like I am getting an infection. If it is from something I ate and my stomach starts getting painful or upset, I immediately reach for the colloidal silver and take two heaping spoonfuls. That usually takes care of it. If not, I take a pill of garlic or even stronger, allicin (a garlic extract) with meals once a day until it clears up. If I feel like I am getting a cold, I start gargling with mouthwash, to keep the infection out of my lungs, then take a combination of Immune Defense from Lifepharm and something called LDM-100 for a few days. I also like a zinc supplement like AirBorne that provides essential minerals as well. If I need more, I add to the protocol high dose vitamin C with a little baking soda and D3 for a few days. If I still need more, I make high strength ginger tea and sip on that for a few days.

If I have a persistent head cold, I take 3 drops of Oregano oil, Frankincense Oil, Myrrh oil, peppermint oil and a couple drops of Eucalyptus Oil in a large pot, pour in boiling water, cover my head with a towel and breath in the steam for a good 10 minutes or so at least once day. If I need more help, I jump under my half-moon IR sauna from Sunlighten, and get a "fever" going by raising my body temperature. A fever mobilizes the immune system to help it do its job. Plus sweating out toxins never hurts.

I have been taking Beta 3D Glucan from Better Way Health for years as one of the best proven Beta Glucan sources on the market to boost my immune system, but it is very expensive. Once a year, around the end of November, they run a half-price sale, so that is when I stock up for the year. I have been reading some very good clinical studies on EpiCor lately and how it acts in four ways to keep your immune system healthy, including but not limited to supplying Beta Glucan, as it is a fermented yeast product, using the same yeast as Better Way Health. There are many companies that produce formulas using EpiCor in various combinations and they may all help. Dr. Mercola just came out with one, too. I will probably give it a try and keep some on hand for that nasty infection that comes around. But I take Better Way Health year-round, as a preventative measure.

For really tough sinus infections, start with a couple of sprays of XLEAR, a Xylitol spray that helps break up biofilm, a film that microbes secrete to keep them from being destroyed by the immune system. Then I get out my Nettie Pot, put sea salt and combination of essential oils in it, usually a couple of drops of frankincense and oregano, but will change it up if I need more to wipe out the infection. Experiment with your essential oils until it wipes out the infection. Then I fill the pot with warm water and flush out my sinuses morning and night. Sometimes, this is the only way to get rid of a sinus infection that no doctors can touch.

You can experiment with any of these natural remedies or many others to see what works best for you to keep your illness under control and expedite healing. I take Beta Glucan five days week to keep my immune system in fairly good condition. Remember, the body is designed to get sick and recover. That is how our immune system works, so you mostly need to give the body what it needs in increased amounts (the body's use of essential vitamins and minerals vastly increases during times of illness) to help it fight the infection.

If you are in very poor health or are immune compromised, that is when you may need medical help. If you are not getting better in a reasonable time, it is time seek medical attention. Or if you see some weird symptoms that seem odd or unusual to you, get it checked out. It could save you lots of suffering.

And don't forget, stress lowers immunity making you susceptible to all sorts of infection and cancer. So, work hard on meditation, spending time with family and friends, exercise, relaxation, fun, sleep, yoga, Tai Chee, Tapping (Emotional Freedom Technique) to deal with old pent up negative energy (Google Nick Ortner) or do whatever it takes to lower stress levels in your life. This is really important!!

CHAPTER 14

Anti-Aging Philosophy and Hacks

This is going to be a wide-ranging chapter because, the fact is, everything in this book is about slowing down aging and living to your maximum potential while on this planet. After I review the basics of helping you live a healthy life, I go into some of the details of the latest science and research into things you can try to extend your life beyond world-wide average life spans. Personally, I do not want to live longer than my brain or body can tolerate. In other words, being wheel chair bound and mentally non-functional is not what I call living. So, it is important to not only extend years but also functionality along with it.

So, why do we age and is there anything we can do about it? This is a very complicated question. For example, at almost the highest level, there are 7 basic theories on why we age (information obtained from GreenMedInfo.com.)

1. THE RATE OF LIVING THEORY

Although no longer accepted by modern day scientists, perhaps the oldest explanation of aging is the rate of living theory.

Ancient philosophers believed we possess a finite amount of some "vital substance"—for example, a predetermined number of breaths or heartbeats. When that substance runs out, it's the end of the line.

2. THE EVOLUTIONARY SENESCENCE THEORY

Evolution does not seem to be favored by aging, so this theory focuses on the failure of natural selection to affect late-life traits. The term "senescence" refers to deterioration with age. Certain undesirable genes and mutations do not express their harmful effects until later in life. These cannot be selectively eliminated when passed on to future generations because they don't express themselves until the reproductive years are over. In other words, natural selection—because it operates via reproduction—can have little effect on later life. These undesirable genes cannot be eliminated through natural selection and result in aging.

3. THE CROSS-LINKING/GLYCATION HYPOTHESIS

This theory is based on the observation that our body's proteins and other structural molecules tend to develop dysfunctional attachments as we age—they form cross linkages to one another. These inappropriate links or bonds cause problems by reducing the mobility or elasticity of proteins and other molecules. Some research suggests crosslinking is the mechanism for aging. You might be familiar with the term "glycation." Glycation or glycosylation is one of the main ways crosslinking occurs. Glucose molecules can stick to proteins and transform them into brownish molecules called advanced glycosylation end products (AGEs). These molecules interfere with and disable the proteins' functions. Glycation is what causes food to brown when cooked. Additionally, evidence suggests glycation contributes to the formation of beta-amyloid, the protein found clumped together in the brains of Alzheimer's patients.

4. THE GENOME MAINTENANCE HYPOTHESIS

This theory proposes DNA damage and gene mutations as the mechanism for aging. Damage caused by oxidative free radicals, mistakes in replication, or outside environmental factors such as radiation or toxins are part of everyday life. Resulting mutations occurring in our egg or sperm cells can be passed on to future generations, whereas those occurring in other types of cells cannot be passed on. Our bodies have repair mechanisms to correct most of these disadvantageous mutations, but those that persist will accumulate and eventually cause cells to malfunction and die, resulting in aging. Because a large proportion of free radicals comes from normal cellular energy production, this theory has particular implications for our mitochondria (intercellular powerhouses). Mutations in mitochondrial DNA accumulate with age and are associated with a decline in mitochondrial function. Many scientists believe that mitochondrial aging is an important contributor to overall aging.

5. THE OXIDATIVE DAMAGE/FREE RADICAL HYPOTHESIS

This theory suggests that aging is caused by oxidative damage by free radicals. Free radicals are toxic byproducts from normal cell metabolism. Antioxidants neutralize many of these free radicals, but those that persist can damage DNA, proteins, and mitochondria. Oxidative damage accumulating over time causes aging and age-related diseases. As with the Genome Maintenance Hypothesis, mitochondria play a central role. More than 90 percent of a cell's free radicals are produced in the mitochondria, so they are at particularly vulnerable to damage. This creates a self-perpetuating cycle in which oxidative damage impairs mitochondrial function, which results in the propagation of even more free radicals. Although mitochondria have some capacity to repair their DNA, the mechanisms are not as effective as those used by the cell to repair nuclear DNA and deteriorate over time. Eventually, mitochondrial damage leads to apoptosis, or cell suicide.

6. THE NEUROENDOCRINE HYPOTHESIS

This theory ties aging to the deterioration of hormone function. As we age, the connections between our brain and endocrine system become dysfunctional, leading to a variety of problems such as high blood pressure, impaired sugar metabolism, and sleep abnormalities, muscle mass loss. A flood of recent evidence points to one hormone pathway in particular: IGF-1 (insulin growth factor-1). IGF is activated by human growth hormone. Higher IGF-1 levels are associated with shorter life expectancy. Interestingly, this flies in the face of popular support for anti-aging treatments involving growth hormone injections, which increase circulating IGF-1. Rather than extending life, growth hormone treatment may actually do the opposite. A recent study found that people who genetically lack an ability to use growth hormone enjoy a lower risk of both cancer and Type 2 diabetes.

7. THE REPLICATIVE SENESCENCE HYPOTHESIS

This theory of aging has to do with cell division and telomeres. Think of telomeres as the protective "end caps" on chromosomes. The theory is that repeated cell division leads to shortened telomeres, and short telomeres are associated with faster aging, therefore shortened lifespan. When telomeres become short they can break, leading to a variety of age-related diseases and conditions. Many human cells have a limited capacity to reproduce themselves. Most scientists believe the limiting factor is the length of the cell's telomeres. Each time a cell divides, it must first double its chromosomes so that each daughter cell receives a full complement of genetic material. Each division results in the loss of a small bit of the chromosomes' telomeres. After about 40 to 60 divisions, the telomeres reach a critically short length such that the cell can no longer replicate and stops dividing. These cells become "senescent" in the sense that, although they don't die, they can no longer reproduce. For quite some time, scientists viewed telomeres as a sort of "cellular clock" that might hold the key to aging, but the thinking now is that while telomeres may contribute to aging, they do not govern it. They are merely one piece of the puzzle. In humans, not all types of tissue contain actively replicating cells—brain and heart, for example. Telomere shortening is not universal among species.

Besides these more detailed theories, one can still ask a question at a higher of level of thinking, like: so why are we designed to age. If it is a particular gene, why do we have that gene in the first place? Or if it is a slow accumulation of destructive products that cause more and more damage to our DNA, why don't our bodies repair the damage more effectively? If it is a vital substance or energy that we run out of, why don't we have an unlimited supply? Besides considering divine intentions, if we look at answers to these questions, can it be that somethings in our environment and lifestyle choices at least have an influence in these destructive forces? I always try and back things up and get at the root cause of the issue. Was there sometime in our past several million years history here on earth, when we perhaps lived in the hundreds of years and something changed on earth or solar system or viral/bacterial/plant transfer of genes to cause a genetic or environmental shift leading to shorter lifetimes? These are questions that bounce around in my brain and in the minds of age researchers around the world.

But excluding how we got into this predicament of an incurable disease (aging), how can we deal with the cards we have and reverse or mitigate these seven potential causes, figure out which one (or more) is really causing aging and work that angle, or option 2; ignore all that completely and rejuvenate all the downstream destructive effects of aging (muscle loss, protein damage, bone loss, immune dysfunctions, digestive power loss, cardio-vascular/circulation loss, cognitive decline, joint degeneration, mitochondria function loss, hormonal and metabolism degradation, etc.)

Rejuvenation science is in full steam ahead mode right now (look at the SENS Research Foundation, the home of the famous Aubrey DeGray. There are many more working this angle). The third option is to optimize our life span to our genetic potential. In other words, are we dying early (around age 80) simply because we are not taking the best care of ourselves and our environment? How long and healthy could the average person expect to live if we all did everything right in terms of a healthy lifestyle, nutrition protocol and fixing the environmental toxin issue? To answer that question, we would first have to know what "everything right" is, right? And that is what modern nutrition science is all about, helping us figure out how to live as long as possible under the current genetic restrictions.

Could we all live to 120 if we did everything right? Perhaps. We don't know. Why don't we know? Because, the science is so new that no one who is adopting and living according to all the healthy science these days, is old enough to prove out the science. The fourth option is to biohack your way into a longer life, similar to option 2, using the best biochemical knowledge combined with strategies like calorie restriction, mitochondria support supplements, anti-inflammatory compounds, immune boosting protocols, ketosis strategies, superfoods, herbs and spices, exercise science, hyperbaric treatments, thermal/light treatments, low level electric stimulation, epigenetic interventions, stem cell/blood treatments, and many more to extend lifespans. The fifth option is to accept our average lifespan as it is between 77 and 83 and work on health span, that is, stay healthy and fully functional until the day we pass, with no chronic disease. In this case, our system reaches a magic age, say around the mid-80s, where we quickly deteriorate within a couple of weeks and pass on.

It could be a combination of all these options that lead to a vast increase in health and life spans. There is also a concept called the anti-aging escape velocity put forth by Aubrey DeGray. This is where we try and stay alive as long as possible to allow for time for science to come up with the next big thing to extend it even further in an endless cycle until the point where we just never die.

But first a special mention of mitochondria and accumulating DNA damage as mentioned in options 4 and 5. Some researchers believe the key to life extension is healthy mitochondria. Why, because these produce the energy for our body, and without energy, we cannot function. And as it turns out Mitochondria have their own DNA. Mitochondrial DNA (mtDNA) gets mutations much faster than the DNA in the nucleus. One reason for this is thought to be the presence of ROS or "reactive oxygen species" (also known as "free radicals") in the mitochondria. When mitochondria make energy for us, they create ROS that can damage nearby mtDNA. In fact, this might be the reason why eating less leads to longer lives in animals -- less food, fewer ROS.

The idea is that as mtDNA becomes more and more damaged, the mitochondria cannot produce energy as well and become dysfunctional. This could lead to aging, disease and ultimately, death. Is there any way to test this idea directly? The most direct way to test this hypothesis would be to increase the rate of mtDNA mutations and see if it results in an increased rate of aging. This is exactly the experiment done by a group of researchers in Sweden.

The researchers mutated a gene in mice so that the mtDNA would get more mutations faster. (The way they did this was to modify the enzyme that copies mtDNA, DNA polymerase-g, so that it made more mistakes as it copied mtDNA. The end result of this is that over time, more mutations accumulate.) As expected, the mutant mice had more mutations in their mtDNA. Did they age faster than normal mice? Yes. At about 25 weeks of age the mutant mice started to display signs of aging that are normally seen in much older mice. The mutant mice lived for less than a year instead of for two to three years. So, obviously mutations in mtDNA are part of the aging process. Are they everything? Probably not but they are clearly an important part of the puzzle.

The truth is millions of people die of completely preventable causes, thus lowering average expected age limits and degrading health span. In fact, this may be the first generation of children that are not expected to exceed the age of their parents. In the past, infectious disease killed many of us, significantly lowering average age limit. Now, it is chronic long-term conditions causing diseases such as heart attack, cancer, diabetes, COPD, inflammation, medical error, liver and kidney failure, overwhelming drug resistant infections, blood sepsis or infection, dementia…all these kill millions every year and most are a result of lifestyle choices. But as mentioned in one of the Dots, anti-biotic resistant bad bacteria are coming back to haunt us, killing thousands around the globe every year.

Make sure and read the chapter on natural anti-biotics. Simply addressing gut health which effects so many other body systems and brain functions would go a long way to increasing average life span. Nutrient depletion and lack of vitamins, minerals and plant compounds in our diet weakens our systems and makes us vulnerable to cancer and infections and bone density issues, thyroid failure, enzyme depletion and accelerating aging. Heated, rancid and oxidized oils in almost everything we eat reduce cellular vitality and lower energy reserves.

High dependence on sugar dwarfs our body's capability to stay balanced and destroys our metabolism leading to obesity, diabetes, heart attacks, inflammation, kidney failure and genetic and nerve damage. Lack of exercise leads to weakness, circulation problems, poor brain function, bad hormone creation and circulation, poor immune function, weak hearts, poor insulin sensitivity, degrading muscle mass, increased blood pressure, weak bones, all leading to earlier death. Social and job-related stress causes genetic damage, excessive cortisol, adrenal fatigue, inflammation, immune deficiency, tissue damage and frailty leading to accelerated aging, heart attacks, increased infections and organ failure.

Poor sun exposure leads to vitamin D deficiency and a host of problems. Lack of proper sleep is a critical factor in obesity and poor hormone production, lymph circulation, increased stress and energy depletion. Lack of fiber in your diet leads to bacterial imbalances and infections, increased blood sugar spikes, opening you up to auto Immune conditions, insulin resistance, brain health issues, cancer and poor nutrient absorption. Eating non-GMO and Organic whole foods can protect from environmental toxins, keeping your cells healthier and living without disease. Building fun and relaxation into your life can lower stress and put you more into a healing mode than a tear down mode.

Dealing with past emotional issues and negative emotions can get the intensity down so you are not carrying around that terrible burden for the rest of your life, a burden that leads to your own degraded health. Including lots of antioxidants in your diet can slow down oxidative damage to your DNA, improve heart and circulatory health, reducing heart attack risk and a host of inflammatory conditions. Understanding your food sensitivities that can inflame the body and organs that can lead to early death and eliminating those foods from your diet can allow your body to heal and revitalize your immune system. Exposure to heavy metals and environmental toxins and molds leads to disease and unnecessary suffering.

Bad oral health can lead to heart and lung failures, not to mention heavy metal poisoning and poor digestion. Healing the gut, removing molds from the environment, getting off wheat, taking pro and prebiotics, multivitamin/mineral supplementation can all help with Auto Immune diseases that ravage the body organs by your immune system attacking itself. Good hydration with clean filtered water can make a world of difference in your health. Try drinking six ounces every hour from a metal container, stopping around 6:00 pm every night and see how you feel after a few weeks. You will never go back to being dehydrated again.

These are all lifestyle issues. Attacking these, even one at a time, can significantly improve your health span and get you to your genetic potential of lifespan as a healthy and functioning human being.

But, you say, I am not satisfied with just being healthy. I want to do something extra to stay on top of my game and live longer. What can I do? Here are additional healing protocols, some we have known for years.

- **Vibration/Rebounding**: Helps circulate the lymph in your body and build bone strength, thus strengthening the immune system, brain health and gut health. The better the immune system, the less disease you will have.
- **Detoxing/Colon Cleansing**: Due to unavoidable exposure to toxins, organ cleansing should be a normal practice for all of us. Focus on the colon, liver and gall

bladder. They are key to overall health. There are many strategies and detox protocols, too numerous to mention, but a good start is a monthly coffee enema and an annual liver/gall bladder oil/citrus flush. You can find the details with your friend Google. There are also many herbal and vegetable detoxes as well. Start trying some and see how you feel. Also, an annual heavy metal detox is very good for you. There are many good chelators on the market now along with charcoal binders. Doing both a chelator with a charcoal binder at the same time is very good for you. Dr. Pompa is a very source for good information on true cellular detoxification. Weekly sweating is also a great way to detox and shed heavy metals.

- **Fasting**: Calorie reduction is a great way to clean up old proteins in the body and increase ketones in the blood stream, leading to a host of improvements in overall health. Start with intermittent fasting, skipping breakfast two or three times a week. You can add coconut oil to your coffee in the morning on fasting days to get you through your fast and increase ketones in your bloodstream, or just buy MCT oil or a product called Brain Octane, all of which quickly convert to ketone bodies, but Brain Octane converts quicker than the others. Increased ketones have been shown to have many beneficial effects on cellular metabolism and genetic repair. Plus, increased ketones lower and stabilize insulin levels.

Insulin itself at high levels is extremely toxic to the body in many ways as mentioned earlier. As a matter of fact, it is the number two association with Alzheimer's. Number one is a genetic indicator, ApoA4 and number three is age. This is huge and means that you can get Alzheimer's at any age if your fasting insulin remains too high. One of the best Podcasts on Ketosis and the biochemistry involved with sugar and fat metabolism is hosted by Mike Mutzel. It is called High Intensity Health. I highly recommend listening to it.

And, a nice full-day water fast, dinner to dinner once a week or so, is really good, if it does not stress you out too much. Protein restriction through fasting brings on a state of autophagy, a self-cleaning cellular mechanism that cleans out toxic cellular debris. Most research says that autophagy starts at about the 12-hour point in your fast. So, if you stop eating at say 8 pm, skip breakfast and then have your first meal at 12 pm, that is 16 hours of fasting, plenty of time to kick in the self-cleaning process. It also helps with sugar control in that you keep your insulin levels low during the fasting period (sugar causes insulin spikes), thus helping to lower insulin resistance.

Insulin resistance is one of the prime markers of Type 2 Diabetes. Plus, Insulin itself at high levels is extremely toxic to the body in many ways. As a matter of fact, it is the number two association with Alzheimer's. Number one is a genetic indicator, ApoE4 and number three is age. This is huge and means that you can get Alzheimer's at any age if your fasting insulin remains too high. One of the best podcasts on ketosis and the biochemistry involved with sugar and fat metabolism is hosted by Mike Mutzel. It is called High Intensity Health. I highly recommend listening to it.

- **Vitamin/mineral Supplementation:** Vitamins/minerals can be lacking in your normal diet, especially these days with depleted soils and western processed foods. Supplementation may be the only way to get and fulfill your body's daily requirements.

- **Morning Start:** First thing in morning, start with a little hot water, add 4 drops of iodine, magnesium salts, MSM (Sulphur), half a lemon of juice, a little local raw honey and cayenne pepper and drink it down. It tastes fine and has many good cleansing and circulation effects on the body, while providing key minerals your body requires for daily operation.
- **Meditation/Prayer:** These put you in parasympathetic mode which helps the body rebuild. Our lives today are filled with stress so any quiet time where you can go inwards, find your center and connect to a greater whole, can help balance your body and allow complete rebuilding to take place. Further, it strengthens the immune system. We know now that bad stress lowers immunity, making you susceptible to all kinds of infections and cancer.
- **Breath Work:** breathing properly is a good way to enter a meditative state or just simply to relax before, during and after a stressful day. We know now that stress lowers the immune system, which can lead to increased infections and cancer, so it is good to keep your stress under control by meditation and breath work. Try box breathing, breathing in, holding, breathing out, holding; all to a count of 5 for each leg in the box.
- **Fermented Products:** making your own fermented vegetables/drinks have been shown to add much needed bacterial content to your gut. You cannot live without an abundance of good bacteria in your gut. These are probiotics. There are also foods called prebiotics that feed those good bacteria in the form of fiber and resistant starches. Increasing fiber content and consuming fiber each day is critical to a healthy intestinal tract. The good gut bacteria crowd out the bad ones, helping to prevent gut infection and a host of gut diseases.

- **Weight Control:** Obesity is unhealthy so keeping your weight down through calorie restriction and other methods is known to extend lives and keep you functioning well.

  So, you say, "I want to live to until I am 120 or beyond." Well, then you need to try some of the latest anti-aging strategies that science has uncovered, and they seem to be endless. Will they definitely work? Well, we don't know because while we have been able to extend lives of animals or microbes in the labs, or have seen results from looking at and measuring certain biomarkers with these strategies, or have seen remarkable healing in this part of the body or another part, this is new science, so we have no evidence on humans who have tried them all or some and have lived to 120 or beyond because of these strategies. But I can tell you this, we are seeing remarkable results in limited studies, labs and some human trials, especially with Stem Cells. So, let's start there.

- **Stem Cell Treatments.** Stem cells are not a new discovery, but their potential for healing has recently gained a great deal of attention in the realm of regenerative medicine. More people are discovering that their joints need support to hold up to their activity level, and athletes are looking for non-surgical methods to keep them active. Instead of signing up for multiple joint replacements, stem cell treatment appears promising.

  Experiencing joint pain doesn't automatically mean that a joint replacement is necessary. Many causes for joint pain never require surgery. The use of stem cells in medicine has advanced greatly in the last few decades. Stem cells are capable of long-term division, thus renewing themselves and replenishing other cells. Stem cells arc also multipotent, meaning they have the potential to work with many types of cells in the body. When applied to a site of injury, the cells utilize the body's innate healing mechanisms to initiate their regenerative action. These properties give stem cell treatment an immense therapeutic capacity. Stem cell injection therapy is performed as a simple in-office procedure. Since stem cells contain natural growth factors, they have the power to do more than just heal damage. They have been found to reduce pain and stiffness and improve mobility.

Many patients start experiencing better overall functionality with just one treatment. Furthermore, the incidence of adverse reaction is very low, because the cells are derived from biological components that already exist in the human body. The future of regenerative medicine has never been brighter. Embryonic stem cell research or using your own stem cells has been going on for decades, but the full potential of these cells is still to be discovered. Stem cells are becoming one of the most-researched areas of medicine, particularly for the knees and hips but for many other applications as well, such as COPD and brain issues. Early research in animals has been encouraging and human studies suggest promising effects.

- **NAD Precursor Supplementation**. NAD is a vital compound for many biological processes in the body, including energy production in your cells and healthy mitochondria. It is well known that it decreases with age. You can take NAD orally now under the tongue or take NAD building blocks. One is now available over the counter in the form of Nicotinamide Riboside or NR. One recent nicotinamide riboside study concluded that taking nicotinamide riboside as an oral supplement, "resulted in a remarkable induction of mitochondrial biogenesis and oxidative metabolism, with an increase in mitochondrial mass."

Once you skip past all the science-y stuff, what does that actually mean? Well, the mitochondria is directly linked to aging. As our bodies age, our mitochondrial production – and functionality – declines. This leads to a wide range of degenerative diseases and ultimately makes us look and feel older. By promoting mitochondrial biogenesis, nicotinamide riboside may be able to "kickstart" the body's anti-aging processes in a way that no other chemical compound can. That means you look, feel, and think younger.

- **Epigenetic Deficiency Supplementation.** Another form of reason 4, we know now that various tags on our genes either hide or promote gene expression. These tags are produced in our bodies through certain processes controlled by certain genes. If you are missing or deficient in these genes, then your genetic tags will be reduced, causing different deficiencies in your health. If you are suffering from some unknown causes, it could well be your epigentics. In that case, you need some genetic testing done to find your genetic abnormalities (SNPs) and start supplementing with the compounds you are missing. This takes an experienced epigenetic practitioner but is well worth the time and money to get you back to good health. One theory on aging says that our epigenetic tags change over our lifetime in a pre-programmed fashion like a timed clock, causing the expression/hiding of age genes, leading to death of the organism. If we can change that process with targeted tag adjustment, or prevention strategies that keep youthful tags in place (prevent DNA damage) we could live forever.

- **Resveratrol.** Resveratrol is part of a group of compounds called polyphenols. They're thought to act like antioxidants, protecting the body against damage that can put you at higher risk for things like cancer and heart disease. It's in the skin of red grapes, but you can also find it in peanuts and berries. Manufacturers have tried to capitalize on its powers by selling resveratrol supplements. Most resveratrol capsules sold in the U.S. contain extracts from an Asian plant called *Polygonum cuspidatum*. Other resveratrol supplements are made from red wine or red grape extracts. Ads touting these supplements on the Internet promise everything from weight loss to a healthier, longer life. Do resveratrol supplements really deliver on those promises? It's gained a lot of attention for its reported anti-aging and disease-fighting powers.

  Still, it's important to note that while experts agree that it does have potential, there's still not enough data to confirm its effectiveness. Still, early research does suggest it might help protect you against: **Heart disease:** It's thought to help reduce inflammation, lower LDL or "bad" cholesterol, and make it more difficult for clots to form that can lead to a heart attack. **Cancer:** It could limit the spread of cancer cells and start killing them. **Alzheimer's:** It may protect nerve cells from damage and fight the plaque buildup that can lead to the disease. **Diabetes:** Resveratrol helps prevent insulin resistance, a condition in which the body becomes less sensitive to the blood sugar-lowering hormone insulin. The condition can lead to diabetes. Researchers believe that resveratrol activates the SIRT1 gene. That gene is believed to protect the body against the effects of obesity and the diseases of aging.
- **IV Cocktails.** There are many varieties and mixtures for IV infusions touting everything from anti-aging to cell repair,

Immune system boosts, anti-viral effects, migraine elimination, hydration, glutathione (our prime anti-oxidant) detoxing, and many others. People have testified they feel wonderful for days after the infusions. I know of no study that has measured the benefits, but it does make sense that bypassing the stomach and intestinal barriers to absorption of vitamins and minerals by injecting them directly into the blood stream would be beneficial to some degree. High dose IV Vitamin C has helped with many disease conditions.

- **Ketosis.** Burning ketone bodies derived from fats instead of glucose for fuel could have many anti-aging effects on the body. Some researchers say that is how we were meant to supply our energy machine and that we should all convert over to fat burning 100 percent of the time. There is intense research going on in this area now and I am watching the results. It is very impressive so far. But, I am also very concerned that people will go too far and stop eating a balance of good fiber, fruits and vegetables as well, critical components of health, giving you the phytonutrients your body needs for long term health. There are certain compounds you cannot get from fat, so we have to be careful and analytical about our food consumption, making sure we supply the body everything it needs. Therefore, I am still recommending an intermittent strategy, going in and out of ketosis, say every other day, for most people, until the science gets better, and we can insure people have the right balance of fat and nutrition in their overall food consumption. Also, keep in mind that fat can escort toxins from bad bacteria into your body (called Lypopolysacharides or LPS). LPS is highly inflammatory. So, if you have gut health problems, get your LPS levels tested and heal that first. Heal the gut lining and get your good bacteria way out numbering your bad bacteria before you go on a high fat diet. A great reference for learning all about Ketosis is: *The Ketogenic Bible* by Dr, Jacob Wilson & Ryan Lowery.

- **Blue Light Blocking.** Visible light is that part of the electromagnetic spectrum that is seen as colors: violet, indigo, blue, green, yellow, orange and red. Blue light has a very short wavelength, and so produces a higher amount of energy. Studies suggest that, over time, exposure to the blue end of the light spectrum could cause serious long-term damage to your eyes. Sources of blue light include the sun, digital screens (TVs, computers, laptops, smart phones and tablets), electronic devices, and fluorescent and LED lighting.

  Because they are shorter, these "Blue" or High Energy Visible (HEV) wavelengths flicker more easily than longer, weaker wavelengths. This kind of flickering creates a glare that can reduce visual contrast and affect sharpness and clarity. This flickering and glaring may be one of the reasons for eyestrain, headaches, physical and mental fatigue caused by many hours sitting in front of a computer screen or other electronic device. Our eyes' natural filters do not provide sufficient protection against blue light rays from the sun, let alone the blue light emanating from these devices or from blue light emitted from fluorescent-light tubes.

  Prolonged exposure to blue light may cause retinal damage and contribute to age-related macular degeneration, which can lead to loss of vision. Potential harmful effects from over exposure include: Disruptions to the circadian rhythm, Digital Eyestrain Syndrome: blurry vision, dry and irritated eyes, headaches, neck and back pain, greater risk of certain types of cancers, diabetes, heart disease, and obesity, depression, or permanent eye damage and contribute to age-related macular degeneration. There are many blue light blocking glasses now available to help you lower your exposure and hopefully avoid some of the damaging effects.

- **Collagen Supplementation.** Collagen is one of the most prolific proteins in our body and is the "glue" that holds many of our soft tissues and skin together. As we age, we produce less and less collagen. Supplementation may ease joint pain, reverse skin aging, improve hair, help build muscle and burn fat, reduce cellulite and improve digestive health. Right now, I use Dr. Axe's Collagen and am getting great results.
- **Hormone Supplementation**. As we age, as mentioned in reason 6, hormone levels trail off and balances change, leading to all sorts of aging symptoms. Bio-identical hormone supplementation can help you feel better, stronger and younger again. You should work with a skilled practitioner who can measure your hormone levels and get your system where it needs to be for optimal functioning. Keep in mind that the thyroid controls energy production so if that is off, you are going to feel in terms of reduced energy abundance, but that is just one of the many causes of an overall lack of energy and vitality. It could also easily be a lack of testosterone or other vital hormones that is robbing you of your vitality.
- **Adaptogen Supplementation.** An adaptogen is a natural substance considered to help the body adapt to stress and to exert a normalizing effect upon bodily processes. To qualify as an adaptogen, an herb must be completely safe and non-toxic, it must have broad uses for health, and it must specifically reduce stress, both mental and physical. Remember, stress is a major cause of inflammation and

reduced immune function, two major killers as we age. To put it simply, Adaptogens help you adapt. The following herbs in alphabetical order demonstrate significant adaptogenic activity: Ashwagandha, Eleuthero, Holy Basil, Maca, Ginseng, Rhodiola Rosea, and Schisandra. Regular use of these plants is thought to have numerous health and life extension benefits. They are used heavily around the world, but western civilization has yet to adopt them on a wide basis. There is good science on many of them, but not well known to the public.

- **Red Light Therapy.** The science of light therapy began to gain broader recognition in 2001 when NASA first discovered that red and near infrared light have very strong cellular regenerating effects. These longer wavelengths have been shown to stimulate mitochondrial function in the cells. Effects include: accelerate healing of surface wounds and mouth ulcers, heal broken bones and injured muscle tissue, stimulate new collagen growth for wrinkle reversal and anti-aging treatments, treat arthritis and injured joints, treat allergic rhinitis, stimulate stem cell growth and nerve regenerations, treat certain types of cancer and is being studied for its effect on reversing the symptoms of Parkinson's, Alzheimer's and cognitive decline. Ari Whitten has written an entire e-book on Red Light therapy with recommendations on the best units to buy for in home therapy. I highly recommend this publication, available on Amazon, even though he freely admits he will get compensated for the purchase of the products he recommends.
- **Increasing overall mitochondrial function.** Many of things I have listed increase mitochondrial function, but there are more. Since mitochondrial health is at the core of all other body functions (without energy and genetic

repair, nothing else works), it is a good strategy to keep them healthy and plentiful. Rather than go into all the potential ways to do this, let me recommend a book by Dave Asprey called Head Strong, who recognizes the value of healthy mitochondria.

- **Alternative Cancer protocols and prevention.** See my chapter on cancer. It is hard to live to 120 and beyond if you die from cancer at 65.
- **Immune Senescence** (sorry about the length of this item but there are many interventions that bolster the immune system). As we age, our immune system function deteriorates, leaving us increasingly susceptible to health threats such as cancer, autoimmunity, infections, and chronic inflammation. This process is called immune senescence. Novel and emerging interventions, as described in LifeExtension information, are: Parabiosis – the transfer of young blood into older blood; Granulocyte-colony stimulating factor (G-CSF) is a protein growth factor made by the body that stimulates production of neutrophils in the bone marrow. A G-CSF drug, filgrastim (Neupogen), is used to bolster low neutrophil counts and decrease risk of infection, particularly in some patients undergoing chemotherapy. Filgrastim can also increase the migration of blood-forming stem cells from the bone marrow into circulation; Caloric restriction in animals has been shown to prolong lifespan and delay aging, and to confer a more youthful profile of T cells; The Mediterranean diet has been shown to protect against several age- and inflammation-related conditions including diabetes, atherosclerosis, obesity, cancers, and neurodegenerative diseases.

The Mediterranean diet is primarily characterized by inclusion of olive oil, fruits, vegetables, legumes, whole grains, nuts, and seeds; with moderate amounts of fish, poultry, cheese, yogurt, and eggs; limited inclusion of red meat, cured meat products, and foods rich in refined sugars; and low-to-moderate alcohol intake, usually in the form of red wine consumed with meals; Regular moderate-intensity exercise can strengthen resistance to infection and improve immune system function; Chronic stress causes dysregulation of innate and adaptive immune responses by promoting persistent systemic inflammation and suppressing immune cells. Lack of sleep can weaken immune function and increase susceptibility to respiratory infections, including the common cold, and chronic lack of sleep may be associated with an increased risk of death; The Cistanche deserticola (C. deserticola) plant has been used historically in traditional medicinal systems as a remedy for chronic infections and other illnesses; Reishi (Ganoderma lucidum) is a medicinal mushroom that has been used in Asia for over 2000 years for immune system support; Pu-erh tea, made from select leaves of Camellia sinensis, has a long history of use in ancient Chinese medicine for anti-aging and preventing infections; Enzymatically modified rice bran, a derivative of rice bran, has been shown to enhance the number and function of immune cells, particularly NK cells (Perez-Martinez 2015; Cholujova 2013; Ghoneum, Abedi 2004; Weiskopf 2009). This specially modified rice bran is a source of the immune-enhancing polysaccharide arabinoxylan (Choi 2014), which has been shown to prevent viral infections of the upper respiratory tract in individuals aged 70 to 95 (Maeda 2004); Dehydroepiandrosterone (DHEA) is a steroid hormone that plays a major role in healthy immune system functioning (Buford 2008; Weksler 1993). DHEA levels decline markedly with age. By age 80, DHEA levels fall to 10–20% of their peak values (Kroll 2015; UMMC 2014); Zinc is an essential trace mineral that is critical to healthy immune function. Zinc deficiency is common in older individuals and causes changes in immune function that resemble those seen in immune senescence; Sufficient vitamin E is critical for maintaining efficient immune function. In fact, a variety of animal studies have shown Vitamin E deficiency can trigger immune suppression; Certain Japanese populations have among the longest life expectancies in the world.

Regular consumption of brown seaweed rich in a compound called fucoidan may contribute to their longevity. Studies have shown fucoidan possesses immune-enhancing, anti-inflammatory, antiviral, and anti-tumor properties; Tinospora cordifolia (T. cordifolia), a medicinal herb used in traditional Ayurvedic medicine, has been the subject of considerable scientific research. Several chemical constituents that enhance immune function have been isolated from T. cordifoli; N-acetylcysteine (NAC) is a form of the sulfur-containing amino acid cysteine, which is a precursor of glutathione, an important facilitator in metabolic detoxification (Brosnan 2006; Santus 2014; Millea 2009).

Glutathione plays a critical role in regulating inflammatory responses, particularly in the lungs. It is essential for some immune functions, including proliferation of T-cells and the cell-killing activity of neutrophils and dendritic cells; Andrographis paniculata is a traditional Chinese medicinal plant used to treat infection, colds, fever, and inflammation; Beta-glucans are polysaccharides (carbohydrates) found in the cell walls of bacteria, fungi, grains including oats, and algae.

Beta-glucans are among the active ingredients responsible for the immune modulating benefits of medicinal mushrooms such as reishi; Lactoferrin is an iron-binding protein found in body secretions including breast milk, colostrum, saliva, tears, nasal secretions, and intestinal fluids, as well as in neutrophils. Lactoferrin's antibacterial effects include damaging microbial cell membranes and binding and isolating iron, which is needed by nearly all bacteria to grow and thrive; Vitamin C supports the function of both the innate and adaptive immune systems and plays an important role in the defense against bacteria and viruses. In addition to stimulating immunity, Vitamin C also appears to restrain excessive immune activity, perhaps in part by interfering with the synthesis of inflammatory cytokines; Whey is the liquid separated from the curds during the cheese making process. Products derived from whey have demonstrated immune-modulating properties (Krissansen 2007; Rusu 2009).

Whey protein is especially rich in precursor amino acids involved in the synthesis of glutathione, a powerful free radical scavenger with anti-inflammatory properties; Garlic, well known for its ability to improve cardiovascular risk factors, also has immune-modulating and immunostimulatory properties, as well as anti-tumor effects. Beyond all this, don't forget that excessive stress causes immune suppression, so do your best to do whatever it takes for you to keep stress levels as low as possible through consistent meditation, tai-chi, pre-recorded sounds/videos, like from Holosync or Deepak Chopra/Opra, affirmations or other meditative practices.

- **Cryotherapy (courtesy of an article by Laura Hanly posted on Chillcryo).** The goal is to get cold enough on a regular basis to switch on metabolic activity in your brown adipose tissue (known as BAT). This is a critical component in sparking off the benefits associated with cold exposure therapy. BAT activity generates heat and starts 'burning' your white fat stores (the stuff everyone tries to get rid of) when your core temperature starts dropping. BAT is considered to be an evolutionary insulation mechanism and is found in nearly all mammals.

Babies also have high levels of BAT, most likely because they haven't developed the ability to shiver yet and so need a way of maintaining a warm core temperature. BAT is usually found in areas where it's easy for heat to directly enter the bloodstream, such as the collarbones, spine and around the organs. As we get older, our stores of BAT reduce, and so this intermediate level of regular cold exposure can help regenerate some of those stores. In order to reach this level, you need to be cold enough that you're noticing it, but not so much that you're consistently shivering.

To achieve this, you might sit in a cold room for a few hours at a time. For example, have your office set to a 50- to 60-degree temperature, and don't wear anything more than cotton pants and shirt. You'll be cold, but not iced over. This is where significant BAT formation happens, and just 10 to 14 days of this (plus continuing on with the cold showers) can be enough to increase your stores.

At this stage you also start experiencing a wider range of benefits, including reduced inflammation in joints and muscles, reduced regular fat stores, greater resistance to cold and pain and improved metabolic function in skeletal muscle. These effects can also be amplified with resistant starch. Now that you've progressed through these levels, you're ready to take on the advanced cold exposure techniques.

This is where you get into ice-in-your-clothing, long swims in frozen or near-freezing water, cryotherapy chambers and the direct application of ice to parts of your body. But remember – you'll get the best results if you go through the preliminary levels first. Your metabolism is hormetic, meaning that it is adaptive, responding best to intermittent exposure to a stressor (like cold exposure). The outcomes you get will be better if you build up your thermogenesis practice over time.

There are a few ways you can engage in cold thermogenesis once you get to this stage. You can wear an ice-vest, filled with ice, that sits over key BAT storage areas, along with compression shorts filled with ice if you really want to take it up a level. You can go to cryotherapy tanks, where you stand in a large cylinder for 3 minutes while -240°F air flows all around you. Or you can find your nearest frozen or near-frozen swimming spot and make a daily habit of jumping in for a 20-minute swim. (Just remember to be smart with this. Being careless with the cold can lead to hypothermia, frostbite or cryoburn, which will most likely undo all the benefits you were trying to reap in the first place.)

At this point, you tend to see another increase in the benefits your body is experiencing (particularly in your immunity): heightened norepinephrine production and responsiveness, increased levels of natural killer cells (cytotoxic lymphocytes), cold-induced leukocytosis and granulocytosis. Additionally, you will see improved thyroid and adrenal function, improved hormonal expression and continuing improvements in body composition, cold and pain tolerance, and lowered incidence of lifestyle related diseases like bone density problems (which can also be improved by Vitamin D3, K2 and C supplementation along with certain minerals: boron, silica and magnesium), cancer and cardiovascular issues.

You'll also see greater insulin sensitivity thanks to BAT's high glucose usage and the subsequent release of adinopectin. Plus, cold therapy has a similar effect on mTor pathways to caloric restriction or intermittent fasting: it induces cellular autophagy, which in turn leads to longer cell life.

- **Ozone and UV Blood Irradiation Therapy.** This therapy has been used for years for various diseases, especially to fight infections, both internal to the body and body surfaces. But it has also shown effectiveness in anti-aging by increasing ATP production, decreasing inflammation, increasing DNA repair and increasing oxygen utilization. Check out the YouTube video called, "Johns Hopkins Cardiologist on Ozone Therapy" for a report from a seemingly very credible source on these types of therapies. They are available now from various centers around the country. Or you can order a home unit as well. Just don't breathe in ozone because it can damage your lungs.
- **Hydrogen Water.** This information comes off of the Dr. Mercola website. I have seen many devices that make hydrogen water and things you can buy to make your own hydrogen water at home. I have never tried any hydrogen water so I cannot personally attest to it making you feel better. I advise you to do your research before you give it a try. Tyler W. LeBaron is a world-class expert on molecular hydrogen, who has done research at Nagoya University in Japan, where most of his research started. He's executive director of the Molecular Hydrogen

Institute (MHI), which is a science-based nonprofit under Section 501(c)(3). MHI is focused on advancing the research, education and awareness of hydrogen as a therapeutic medical gas. LeBaron explains:

"To understand how hydrogen works, we need to understand how free radicals work and why they're produced. First, the hydroxyl radical, which is OH neutral with a lone pair electron, is produced in your body through the Fenton reaction. When free radicals get too high, like superoxide radicals, peroxynitrite [or] ionizing radiation, [they] can be converted to hydroxyl radicals ... [Hydroxyl radicals] are damaging because they're so reactive ... When you look at other free radicals [such as] nitric oxide, that's a very important free radical which causes vasodilation. We don't want to neutralize that. We have superoxide radicals [and] other oxidants like hydrogen peroxide — these are all very important. Of course, too much is bad, but having them in the right concentrations and at the right locations is very good for you. We don't want to just neutralize all of those, whereas hydroxyl radicals or peroxynitrite oxidants, we don't want any of them. That Nature Medicine publication specifically showed that hydrogen could act as a therapeutic antioxidant by selectively reducing the cytotoxic oxygen radicals, specifically the hydroxyl radical and to a lesser extent peroxynitrite, without decreasing the other oxidants like hydrogen peroxide or superoxide ... Most other antioxidants are not selective ... [and] that can be problematic ... Hydrogen is selective in that it's only going to decrease or reduce those toxic radicals like the hydroxyl radical.[4]"

"We need free radicals," LeBaron says, *"and studies have shown you can actually suffer from too much*

oxidative stress and too much reductive stress (or not enough oxidative potential) not only in the same body or the same organ, but in the exact same cell. Too much oxidative stress in the cytosol; not enough oxidative power in endoplasmic reticulum. Hydrogen helps to bring everything back to homeostasis."

To learn more about molecular hydrogen, please visit http://www.molecularhydrogeninstitute.com.

Astragalus Root. This is a known herb with longevity properties, known for over 2000 years. An extract of this is called TA-65 and has been shown to extend Telomeres, the end caps of your genes. A lot of people swear by it. But you have to be wealthy or be very dedicated about a large portion of your income to buy a continual supply of TA-65. It is very expensive. Other than that, you can simply add Astragalus root to your diet at some regular, consistent interval.

Heart Rate Variability. Believe it or not, the less regular your heart beats, the better off you are. The consistency of the space or time between beats indicates whether you are in sympathetic or parasympathetic mode. And you need to be in parasympathetic mode most of the time. This will allow your body to rest, heal and rebuild (anabolic) and to have reserve and resilience. This is called heart rate variability. There are many devices on the market that you can buy now to keep tabs on your HRV. Then you can work towards spending as much time as possible in parasympathetic mode. Athletes and high stress jobs/lives need to really watch out this. Our bodies are not made for chronic physical or emotional stress.

C60 and Olive Oil. Take a look at this. It has been shown to extend the life of rats by up to 90 percent! It is not costly and many people are taking this on a routine basis and have been seeing good results. I have no idea if it is safe over the long term or will actually extend lives in humans.

- **Osteoporosis.** Unfortunately, we all start losing bone mass at one percent per year after age 50. Why? We are not sure. There are many possibilities: lowering Hydrochloric Acid levels in the stomach as we age decreasing digestive capacity, decreasing and changing body hormone levels, decreasing intestinal absorption levels, decreasing calcium food levels, decreasing kidney function, increasing inflammation levels, decreased exercise, increased auto-immune levels. All of these can affect bone densities. So for most of us, although not all, it is simply an aging condition, increased perhaps by the drugs we are taking. But it effects some more than others. Osteoporosis is due to an imbalance that occurs (everything in the body is about balance or homeostasis. See my "Laws of Life" section above.) between the bone building cells, osteoblasts, and the bone tear down cells, osteoclasts. We are not sure why the bone tear down cells start exceeding the build-up cells but here is more information on how the whole process works:

  The body maintains very tight control over the calcium circulating in the blood at any given time. The equilibrium is maintained by an elegant interplay of calcium absorbed from the intestines, movement of calcium into and out of the bones, and the kidney's reclamation and excretion of calcium into the urine. If the serum calcium level falls, the parathyroid glands release of PTH into the blood and this signals cells in bone (osteoclasts) to release calcium from the bone surfaces. PTH also signals the kidney to reclaim more calcium before it is excreted in the urine and also stimulates synthesis of the active form of vitamin D. There are at least three hormones intimately involved in the regulation of the level of calcium in the blood: parathyroid hormone (PTH), calcitonin and calcitriol (1, 25 dihydroxyvitamin D, the active form of vitamin D). PTH comes from the parathyroid glands located behind the thyroid gland in the lower part of the neck and calcitonin comes from cells in the thyroid gland, both of which monitor and maintain calcium levels in the blood. The active form of vitamin D is synthesized in the kidney under the control of PTH.

Special cells that reside in the thyroid gland along with thyroid hormone containing cells release another hormone, calcitonin, into the blood. Calcitonin signals osteoclasts to slow down removal of calcium from bone; this action tends to lower levels of blood calcium. Conversely, shutting off calcitonin allows osteoclasts to get back in business to release needed calcium from bone. The PTH system provides long-term, day-to-day regulation of calcium levels by many hormones working in concert. This hormonal "feedback loop" is governed by the parathyroid glands and the calcitonin secreting cells of the thyroid gland by their constant monitoring of the blood calcium levels. The body also has a minute to minute regulation of calcium levels from osteocytes in bone—these cells can instantly release needed calcium or instantly stop releasing calcium depending on immediate needs (too little or too much calcium coming into the bloodstream)

If we are to extend life spans to 120 and beyond, wouldn't we want to have strong bones, so we don't have to worry about falling down or simple moves that would normally be nothing to our underlying bone support structure? A broken hip for the elderly can in many cases lead to a slow decline and death. A fractured rib or vertebrae in your spine can be very painful.

So, without taking drugs that have side effects, how can we safely rebuild strong bones or least stop bone loss? Here are some well-known mitigations:

- **Exercise and movement.** One of the best things you can do is resistance or weight bearing exercise. And there is no age that is too old to get started. Even if it is using body weight for your resistance. Also, whole body vibration is very good. Just standing on a vibrating plate for 15 minutes a day has been shown to help. That is because muscles have weight. And when you jiggle them around, it places forces on your bones, just like you are lifting weights. There are many on the market, but they are not cheap.
- **High food calcium.** Calcium is needed by many functions in your body, not just your bones. If you are not getting a lot through your diet, your bones get cheated. Taking non-ionic calcium straight has been linked to many cardio vascular issues so it is best to increase consumption through leafy greens and high ionic calcium foods like organic Moringa and Algae. Moringa also has tons of other micro nutrients so it is a great addition overall.
- **Hormones.** Women suffer from estrogen loss, men from testosterone loss. So bioidentical hormone supplementation is always an option as we get older.

- **Vitamin D3/K2/C.** These vitamins are critical for the proper absorption and use of calcium in your body. Make sure your D levels are kept above 50. K2 should be taken with D3. Vitamin C strengthens bones in several ways:
  - ✓ It mineralizes the bone and stimulates bone forming cells to grow.
  - ✓ Prevents too much degradation of bone by inhibiting bone absorbing cells.
  - ✓ Dampens oxidative stress, which is what aging is.
  - ✓ Is vital in collagen synthesis.

  When vitamin C is low, just the opposite happens. Bone cells that degrade bone called octeoclasts proliferate, and bone cells that lay down mineral and new bone called osteoblasts are not formed.

  Studies have shown that elderly patients who fractured bones had significantly lower levels of vitamin C in their blood than those who haven't fractured. Bone mineral density- the thing that the tests measure, is higher in those who supplement with vitamin C, independent of estrogen level.
- **Yoga/Tai Chi.** These may not solve your osteoporosis, but they will improve muscle tone, core strength and balance, keeping you from falling and potentially fracturing a bone.
- **Strontium**. Taking strontium has been shown in studies to reverse bone loss. But long-term supplementation has not been shown safe by science and some adverse effects have been noted. I would like to see more studies on it before I can recommend it.
- **Smoking and alcohol.** Both have been linked to increased bone loss.

- **Insufficient protein.** As mentioned above in my protein chapter, low protein and essential amino acids can lead to bone loss, especially for those around 65 or older.
- **Bone broth/bone powders.** Some alternative products offer ground up bone and bone broths. I have not seen the science to back it up, but I don't think it can hurt and may be a good source of bone minerals and other nutrients for the body. Try and stick with grass fed animals.
- **Almonds.** Studies have shown that eating almonds can be better than normal calcium supplements in slowing down bone loss. We order raw non-radiated almonds in 25-pound bags online. Then we soak some in water for at least 24 hours, then dehydrate them and put them in the fridge. They are fantastic!! Also, I make my own almond butter by throwing a bunch in the Vita Mix blender and using the plunger to grind them into a butter at about mid speed. Then put that in a jar and in the fridge.
- **Ionic Calcium.** Take a look at DocofDetox's website on Ionic Calcium. This is late breaking stuff in that normal calcium supplementation has been shown to be dangerous to your health over the long term because it is not in ionic form, that is with a double plus charge on the calcium atom. There is now a company produces this ionic calcium and they say it is safe and getting great results, helping to stimulate the body to restore normal physiology in its calcium balancing systems and thus rebuilding bone density. If this is all true, it may be a great breakthrough for many conditions. It is too new for me to recommend but you may want to check it out. I certainly am.

Also, here is another news flash – bones are endocrine organs!! Your osteoblasts secrete a hormone called osteocyclin. Many studies show a relationship between this hormone and glucose metabolism. Isn't that interesting. As we lose bone mass, we could be affecting our metabolic strength, thereby reducing the amount of energy available to our system for all sorts of body needs. And it could tie bone mass into conditions like diabetes and insulin production and resistance. More research is needed. But, if this effect of osteocylin is confirmed and we can find ways to stay active and slow down bone loss, or put another way, exercises like walking and weight training as we get older may have tremendous effects on available energy through bone density retention. The more we walk and keep muscle mass, the more we keep bone density, the better glucose metabolism we have, the more energy we have…everything is connected…

That is about all I want to say on anti-aging science. The problem is, so far we have not figured out how to stop aging so all we can do is work around it and limit its effects until our bodies finally give out. But perhaps with the current emphasis on anti-aging science, we will actually figure this out and will all truly be able to live a healthy and functional life for 120 years or more. Time will tell, if we live that long.

CHAPTER 15

Cancer

Sometimes, I just want to stand on a mountain top and cry while I scream: come on people…connect the dots…you can prevent or beat your cancer! You just have to educate yourself and then make significant changes in your life. I could easily write an entire book on this area, including western medicine research and standard of care and alternative treatment options for cancer. In fact, many people have. And they have produced video series, coaching classes, webinars, websites, newsletters, alternative treatment clinics and tons of information on the cause(s) and treatment options.

There are tons of video testimonials of people that have beat their cancers, even genetic-based cancers with alternative treatments. I cannot add anything new to the discussion. So, instead of regurgitating some of that, I will simply give you some references to go check out, so you can begin your education on this subject. Many people have "beaten" cancer with alternative treatments either alone or in combination with standard medical care. There is tons of science to show that certain natural compounds fight cancer. I use many of them myself as a prevention strategy. We also know that stress lowers the immune system and the immune system is needed to keep cancer in check.

So, it is logical that if you suffered a severe trauma in your life that is unresolved, or are under tremendous stress for an extended period, your immune system could allow cancer to take hold. Also, since cancer is basically a disease of aging (although there are exceptions), and your immune system deteriorates as we age, we could infer that the unabated growth of cancer is a result of a lowered immune system in most cases. One strategy for cancer prevention would be to do what it takes to keep your immune system strong. But, I would never do just one thing to prevent cancer. In fact, I do many things. Is it enough? Only time will tell. I am 64 now and so far, so good.

Here are some references to get you started:
Book and Video Series: Chris Wark *Beat Cancer*

Book: Bill Henderson's *Beating Cancer Gently*

Book/Video Series/Newsletters/info: Thetruthaboutcancer.com (Ty Bollinger)

Book: *Tripping over the Truth* (Travis Christofferson)

Book: *Cancer Research Secrets* (Dr. Keith Scott-Mumby)

Website: cancertutor.com

Website: Drgreger.org (search for caner related subjects)

GreenMedInfo.com (search for cancer fighting compounds)

Book: *When Cancer Disappears: The Curios Phenomenon of "Unexpected Remission"* (Dr. Kelly Turner)

You Tube: Dr. Buttar: *The Seven Toxcities* and his other books and publications

I hope this is useful to you and that you read some of these to develop your own cancer prevention strategy. If you just want a Health Coach who will show you what to do without all the reading, you can contact me at: bob@conscioushealthclub.com

THOUGHT BREAK #5: I CHOOSE THEREFORE I AM

We live in a relative world. Einstein proved that in physics and relativity theories, but could we extend his thinking a bit further to the soul and spiritual realm? In our physical world, distance and time are relative to the speed with which we are traveling. With our identity and our feelings about ourselves in this relative world, we make our way through life by interacting with our emotional environment, that is, the situations we encounter and the people we interact with. And I guess ultimately, unless you live in nature as a hermit and never see another soul, every situation you encounter is a result of people relating to others- somewhere, somehow.

Within a certain set of boundaries (we probably way underestimate those boundaries, needlessly restricting our options), we appear to have a certain degree of freedom in the choices we make. Those choices are presented to us daily as we go through our lives, growing up, moving through the educational system, entering the workforce, doing our hobbies, making dietary, exercise, lifestyle and relationship choices, budgeting our time, choosing our mates, deciding what is on the agenda for the day, an almost unlimited set of choices.

Perhaps what we don't realize is that these choices create who we are, and in this context, allows us to do what is most endowed to us by the Great Creator; that is, exercise the experience of creation. There is this clear link between these three facets of being: choosing, creating and establishing who we are. In a sense, this gives us control over who we want to be as we go about the Godly work of providing all facets of feelings as an expression of experiencing God's true state of being.

The question comes as to whether these situations that come to us that allow us to choose who we are at any given moment, are random, or do we bring those situations to us by our intent and need to grow? Since we are "creating" beings, do we somehow create those situations through unknown forces in the universe, that present to us the pathway to make the choices we need to make to become the beings we want to be? And is there a combining effect from multiple people with multiple intents, like harmonics, so that not only are you facing your own situations that you created and unknowingly have brought to you, but also situations that harmonics have brought to you, ultimately tying you unavoidably into the entire population of the planet?

If there is inherent joy in creating, and to me there certainly is, then most of us are missing out on the unlimited amounts of joy in our daily lives just because we not mindful of what we are creating or that we are in a constant, unyielding non-stop process of creating. In a sense, a choice is also a creation, in that you are, by your choices, creating who you want to be by the outcome of your choices. We may be creating on at least two levels, 1) creating the situations that confront us, either by our own intent and thoughts or through harmonics with others, and 2) creating ourselves by our choices and the outcomes of those situations.

If this truly was the case, then we could derive joy out of life in this realm no matter what the situation was that presented itself to us, be it good or bad, knowing we are in control of our own journey, shaped by the choices and creations we make. In other words, we could enter a more playful, joyful realm whereby we understand the creative forces in play, and use those forces to create and experiment, seeing what happens when choose one creative path versus another. But, that also puts a tremendous burden on us; a burden some cannot bear. Life would be so much easier if all our hard choices were made for us. Or, if we had some loving hand guiding us throughout our lives, helping us to make the choices that serve us best, that would be good. Maybe that is where love comes in.

When confronted with a choice, a guiding light might be, "What would love do?" or "Which direction would result in a higher version or ourselves?" These seem to be good guideposts. If we were truly walking in wakefulness, mindful of this process at every second of our lives, it would hopefully make our time here truly heaven on earth. That is what I try to do….

CHAPTER 16

Autoimmune Disorders

Some people estimate that as much as 70 percent of the U.S. population are affected by auto immune disorders, where the body attacks its own tissues. This disease can be going on for years (And usually does). That period of increased anti-bodies to a particular tissue is called the Prodromal Period, where you are not experiencing symptoms, but you do have a building condition of increased anti-bodies prior to the onset of symptoms. Auto Immunity is merely a heightened or increased level of a normal level of attack.

You see, we have a normal level of antibodies to all of our tissues in the body, antibodies that help destroy old and dying cells as a normal part of growth and destruction and turnover of our body tissues. As you may know, our body is in a constant state of replacement and we grow and replace each organ/tissue at different rates, some are very fast turn overs in the days and weeks, some are slower in the months and years. Antibodies are there to attack and destroy and remove all this cellular waste and keep our bodies new and clean and operating efficiently.

Problems come when our antibodies start removing tissue faster than we can replace it and then slowly, without our knowledge, we start moving into a situation where that organ function can no longer support minimum body requirements. Since studies have proved that auto immune disease can start years before any symptoms appear, we need to take preventative measures now to stop auto immune diseases later. What really causes this over reaction? We are not sure of the biochemistry but experts in the field believe there are three pillars that excite our tissue antibodies into a frenzy and cause them to multiply and go after our tissues way beyond normal maintenance levels. Where ever you are genetically predisposed to have a problem, antibodies for that particular tissue multiply and attack that particular organ/tissue. It is probably related to an absorption of toxic agents into the tissues of susceptibility, causing an inflammatory reaction, alerting the immune system to build more anti-bodies.

For example, if you build up gluten in your liver or any other organ or tissue, and you have a gluten sensitivity or intolerance, those gluten anti-bodies will go after that tissue and slowly destroy it. We know now that gluten sensitivity can result in attack on any organ or joint/ tissue in the body, even result in various tumors. So, according to Dr. Tom O'Brian, there are three pillars for triggers (or toxins) to the immune system that can cause excessive tissue anti-bodies: 1) food/water, 2) air contaminants, and 3) an imbalance of gut bacteria.

So, let's start with food. Most humans have problems with modern wheat. Not sure why. It could be the gluten in the wheat. Or it could be the lectins in the wheat. Or it could be the stuff they spray on wheat these days to ripen it quicker which contains a deadly chemical called glyphosate. Or it could be that because wheat today has been hybridized literally hundreds of times, more than nature would ever produce itself, we really are eating kind of a franken-wheat, not meant for human consumption.

But several studies have been done now to confirm that most everyone has a bad reaction to modern wheat. Every time we eat wheat, the gut lining suffers and then we heal. But over time, it takes its toll and later in life we can develop all sorts of body issues due to a chronic inflammatory reaction, gluten antibodies or auto immune disease. Other foods can also cause allergic/inflammatory /auto immune reactions. The most common are corn, soy, dairy, peanuts and eggs. So those would be my first picks for elimination to see if you feel better and if your health returns without them for a month or so.

Or it could be that wheat breaks down your barriers and renders you sensitive to hundreds of other foods. For example, if your wheat causes tears in your gut lining, then undigested food of many or all kinds can enter your blood and lymph systems, causing your immune system to go into overdrive with a bunch of "foreign invaders" entering your blood stream and taken up by your tissues. Or, you could just have a genetic sensitivity to some foods. You have to become your own doctor, realize you are not feeling good or thinking well and start eliminating certain foods out of your diet for at least a month and see if you feel better.

Also, GMO's could really be bothering you, destroying your gut lining and allowing harmful toxins into your system, causing an auto immune response. There are two basic types of GMO's: one that modifies genetics of the plant to be able to withstand the weed killer, Round Up, and the main component glyphosate. Here, you get a double whammy, the genetically modified plant (God only knows what that does to you.) and the terrible destruction from the weed killer. On the other type of GMO, the plant is transformed to produce its own pesticide, keeping bugs away. So here, since plants can transfer genetic material into your gut, you could be turning your gut into a pesticide factory. Is that really what you want going on inside you? Corn and soy are almost all GMO these days, so it would be wise to eliminate these or eat organic to eliminate GMOs from your diet.

Of course, now the FDA has approved genetically altered Salmon. I would definitely stay away from that until we know if it is safe. That would take a several years study of human trials to confirm it.

The water we drink could be loaded with toxins or heavy metals. We need to be as careful as possible to drink fresh clean water, hopefully not from a plastic bottle, which carries its own toxins, even if it is BPA-free. It is well worth the money to buy a good water filter.

The second pillar, the air we breathe, makes tons of people sick without knowing it due to mold. And mold can be cross-reactive with gluten meaning, you could be off gluten from wheat and yet still test high for gluten antibodies in your system because the mold proteins in your body look similar to gluten. Toxic mold can be devastating to your health and cognitive functions. So, if you tried the major food eliminations and do not feel better, but do feel better when you leave your house, or miss work for a week, or air out your house, or live or work in a place that has ever been flooded or without air conditioning for some time, then suspect mold and get your house/work place checked for it. There are many ways to get rid of mold from a structure. Some are as simple as spraying. Some require tearing out all the drywall. Some are a lost cause and you simply have to move to regain your sanity. But isn't your health worth it?

The third pillar of causes for auto immune disease is gut health related to gut flora. Bad bacteria in your gut contain a molecule called lypopolysaccharide or LPS, also known as endotoxins. Tears in your gut lining (called leaky gut), allow these into your blood stream and elicit a strong immune response and have long been recognized as a key factor in septic shock. This is serious stuff. Some studies estimate that Sepsis contributes to as many as half of all hospital deaths in the U.S. So naturally, a strong immune reaction to LPS could be causing your antibodies to go into overdrive.

There are many things that can cause leaky gut, like auto immune reactions, food sensitivities, pesticides or overgrowth of bad bacteria. When working with auto immune problems, you must focus on gut bacteria and healing the gut lining. Good prebiotics and probiotics along with fermented foods can help rebalance the gut. Charcoal binders can bind to LPS molecules and keep them out of your blood stream. GAP diets with bone broth can help heal gut linings. Natural antibiotics like allicin and berberine can reduce or eliminate bad bacteria from the upper intestine in case you have Small Intestine Bacterial Overgrowth or SIBO. Be aware that certain fats like palmitic acid in palm oil can escort LPS from your intestines into your blood stream, something you want to stay away from.

High fiber diets can help feed good bacteria and keep you from becoming constipated. A good supply of magnesium every morning (build up to this because if you are not used to taking it, it can be traumatic) is good for the whole body, but also can keep your bowels moving smoothly. Turmeric/curcumin can lower inflammatory reactions as well as Green Tea or green tea extracts. Citrus and olive oil-based liver/gall bladder flushes can get your bile moving again which increase fat digestion and keep your bowels moving, lowering your overall toxic load (contact me if you would like a protocol, and they should be available on line).

If all else fails, go to a functional medicine doctor or naturopath or health coach who understands all this and can get you out of this autoimmune trap you have been in for many years. Some MS patients have gotten out of their wheel chairs by following these and other nutritional protocols (see Dr.Wahl's book). There are tons of autoimmune diseases and the number of people affected are growing all the time. With carcful attention and planning, you can add many years of healthy life to your overall health and life span simply by paying attention to these details.

There may also be a connection to the way you were born. Your gut bacteria train your immune system so if you had a natural child birth, you had an initial inoculation of bacteria from your mother's vaginal wall. However, if you were born by C-section, you missed that great opportunity of an incredible microbe inheritance. Think about it, these bacteria could be ancient, being passed down from generation to generation, potentially going back to the original humans on the planet. These ancient strains may be critical to our health. I find that many of my clients with auto-immune diseases started life at a disadvantage with a C-section delivery. If it was my wife and child undergoing a C-section, I would demand the docs smear vaginal fluid all over my child immediately after delivery.

We need to wise up on auto immunity quickly since it is growing at record pace in the world. The last thing we need is to start destroying our own organs and tissues, enhancing chronic inflammation, lowering fertility, and fostering the number one cause of most diseases and early demise and suffering, inflammation.

CHAPTER 17

Get Tested

Getting tested can be extremely valuable to your health. Besides potentially finding something you need to work on, it gives you a baseline to measure by over the years. Self-quantifiers get tested frequently, even if it comes out of their own pockets. Insurance will pay for annual tests as long as the test is recommended by a physician and it is within the standard of care for that type of treatment. But many times, you can ask for items to be added to your test and sometimes insurance will cover it and sometimes they won't, so you have to be prepared to pay for those additions, just in case.

But what should you ask for as some of the more important additions during your annual physical, if they do not already include them? Here are some of my favorites (I could not say it any better than info provided by Dr. Mercola, so here are his recommendations). Keep in mind, in my view, there are three main levels of testing - this is just the basic level of testing, then we will talk about more advanced testing.

Level 1 Testing

Vitamin D. Optimizing your vitamin D is one of the easiest and least expensive things you can do for your health. My recommendation is to get your vitamin D level tested twice a year, when your level is likely to be at its lowest (midwinter) and highest (midsummer). This is particularly important if you're pregnant or planning a pregnancy, or if you have cancer. Based on the research done and data collected by GrassrootsHealth, 40 ng/mL (100 nm/L) is the cutoff point for sufficiency to prevent a wide range of diseases.

For example, most cancers occur in people with a vitamin D blood level between 10 and 40 ng/mL, and published data suggests a whopping 80 percent of breast cancer recurrences — four out of five — could be prevented simply by optimizing vitamin D and nothing else.

For optimal health and disease prevention, a level between 60 and 80 ng/mL (150 to 200 nm/L) appears to be ideal. While the American Medical Association claims 20 ng/mL is sufficient, research suggests 20 ng/mL is barely adequate for the prevention of osteomalacia, and clearly far too low for other disease prevention or improvement.

Omega-3 Index. Like vitamin D, your Omega-3 level is also a powerful predictor of your all-cause mortality risk and plays a vital role in overall health, especially your heart and brain health. Recent research funded by the National Institutes of Health found having a higher Omega-3 index was associated with a lower risk for cardiovascular events, coronary heart disease events and strokes. Omega-3 also helps improve pain, especially when combined with vitamin D.

(Omega-3 fats are precursors to mediators of inflammation called prostaglandins, which is, in part, how they help reduce pain. Anti-inflammatory painkillers also work by manipulating prostaglandins.) The Omega-3 index is a blood test that measures the amount of EPA and DHA Omega-3 fatty acids in your red blood cell (RBC) membranes. Your index is expressed as a percent of your total RBC fatty acids.

The Omega-3 index reflects your tissue levels of EPA and DHA and has been validated as a stable, long-term marker of your Omega-3 status. An Omega-3 index over eight percent is associated with the lowest risk of death from heart disease. An index below 4 percent puts you at the highest risk of heart disease-related mortality. If you're below eight percent, increase your Omega-3 intake and retest in three to six months.

You can save money by getting the combined vitamin D and Omega-3 index testing kit, offered by GrassrootsHealth as part of its consumer-sponsored research. Your best sources of animal-based Omega-3 are small, cold-water fatty fish such as anchovies, herring and sardines. Wild Alaskan salmon is another good source that is low in mercury and other environmental toxins. These fish are also a decent source of vitamin D, making them doubly beneficial.

If you're not eating these foods on a regular basis, your alternatives include fish oil and krill oil. The latter is my preferred choice, as it contains DHA and EPA in a form that's less prone to oxidation. The fatty acids in krill oil are also bound to phospholipids, which allow the DHA and EPA to travel efficiently into your hepatic system; hence they're more bioavailable. Studies have shown that krill oil may be 48 times more potent than fish oil.

Fasting Insulin. Insulin resistance is a driving factor for virtually all chronic disease, making fasting insulin testing a really important health screen. Any meal high in grain and sugar carbs typically generates a rapid rise in your blood glucose. To compensate, your pancreas secretes insulin into your bloodstream, which lowers your blood sugar. If you did not have insulin to do this, you would go into a hyperglycemic coma and die.

Insulin, however, will also catalyze the conversion of excess sugar into fat cells. Typically, the more insulin you make, the fatter you become. If you consistently consume a high-sugar, high-grain diet, your blood glucose level will be correspondingly high and over time your body becomes desensitized to insulin, requiring more and more insulin to get the job done.

Eventually, you become insulin resistant and prone to weight gain, then prediabetic, and then you enter full-blown diabetes. Prediabetes is defined as an elevation in blood glucose over 100 mg/dL but lower than 125 mg/dl, at which point it formally becomes Type 2 diabetes. However, any fasting blood sugar regularly over 90 mg/dL is really suggestive of insulin resistance, and the seminal work of the late Dr. Joseph Kraft suggests 80 percent — 8 out of 10 — Americans are in fact insulin resistant. Although he recommended an oral glucose tolerance test, which also measures insulin, this is a far more challenging test, and for most a fasting insulin test will suffice.

The fasting blood insulin test is far better than a fasting glucose test as it reflects how healthy your blood glucose levels are over time. It's important to realize it's possible to have low fasting glucose but still have a significantly elevated insulin level. And yes, it must be fasting for at least eight hours, otherwise the results are nearly meaningless. A normal fasting blood insulin level is below 5, but ideally, you'll want it below 3. If your insulin level is higher than 3 to 5, the most effective way to optimize it is to reduce or eliminate all forms of dietary sugar. Intermittent fasting, partial fasting and/or water fasting are also effective, and intermittent fasting combined with a ketogenic diet appears to be the most aggressively effective of all.

A ferritin test is a laboratory blood test that measures the amount of ferritin in your blood. Ferritin is the major iron storage protein in your body, so the ferritin test is ordered as an indirect way to measure the iron stores in your body.

Serum Ferritin. For adults, I strongly recommend getting a serum ferritin test on an annual basis, as iron overload can be every bit as dangerous as vitamin D deficiency. While iron is necessary for biological function, when you get too much, it can do tremendous harm by increasing oxidative stress. When iron reacts with hydrogen peroxide, typically in your mitochondria, dangerous hydroxyl free radicals are formed. These are among the most damaging free radicals known and are highly reactive and can damage DNA, cell membranes and proteins. They contribute to mitochondrial dysfunction, which in turn is at the heart of most chronic degenerative diseases.

Unfortunately, the first thing people think about when they hear "iron" is anemia, or iron deficiency, not realizing that iron overload is actually a more common problem, and far more dangerous. Virtually all adult men and postmenopausal women are at risk for iron overload since they do not lose blood on a regular basis and since humans are not at all designed to excrete excess iron, it is simply stored for a rainy day when you might need extra iron from some type of trauma resulting in blood loss.

There's also an inherited disease, hemochromatosis, which causes your body to accumulate excessive and dangerously damaging levels of iron. If left untreated, high iron can contribute to cancer, heart disease, diabetes, neurodegenerative diseases and many other health problems, including gouty arthritis. As with many other lab tests, the "normal" range for serum ferritin is far from ideal. A level of 200 to 300 ng/mL falls within the normal range for women and men respectively, but if you're in this range, know you're virtually guaranteed to develop some sort of health problem.

An ideal level for adult men and non-menstruating women is actually somewhere between 30 and 40 ng/mL. (You do not want to be below 20 ng/mL or much above 40 ng/mL.) The most commonly used threshold for iron deficiency in clinical studies is

12 to 15 ng/mL. You may also consider doing a gamma-glutamyl transpeptidase (sometimes called gamma-glutamyltransferase or GGT) test. GGT is a liver enzyme correlated with iron toxicity and all-cause mortality. Not only will the GGT test tell you if you have liver damage, it's also an excellent marker for excess free iron and is a great indicator of your sudden cardiac death risk.

In recent years, scientists have discovered GGT is highly interactive with iron, and when serum ferritin and GGT are both high, you are at significantly increased risk of chronic health problems, because then you have a combination of free iron, which is highly toxic, and iron storage to keep that toxicity going. To learn more, see "Serum Ferritin and GGT — Two Potent Health Indicators You Need to Know."

High-Sensitivity C-Reactive Protein (hs-CRP). The hs-CRP is a highly sensitive test that measures a liver protein produced in response to inflammation in your body, and chronic inflammation is a hallmark of most chronic diseases. The lower your level the better. Goal would be to be below 0.7 mg/dl. I like to keep mine under 0.2 mg/dl.

Conventional medicine will typically treat underlying inflammation with nonsteroidal anti-inflammatory drugs or corticosteroids. Patients with normal cholesterol but elevated CRP are also frequently prescribed a statin drug. None of these drug treatments address the underlying cause of the inflammation and can do more harm than good in the long run.

Eating a healthy diet low in added sugars and higher in healthy fats, optimizing your vitamin D and Omega-3, lowering your insulin level and exercising on a regular basis will all help to address chronic inflammation. Certain herbs and supplements can also be useful, including astaxanthin, boswellia, bromelain, ginger, resveratrol, evening primrose and curcumin.

One drug option that is both safe and effective is low-dose naltrexone. Naltrexone is an opiate antagonist, originally developed for the treatment of opioid addiction. However, when takin at very low doses, it triggers endorphin production, which helps boost immune function, and has anti-inflammatory effects on the central nervous system.

RBC Magnesium. Magnesium deficiency is extremely common, and recent research shows even subclinical deficiency can jeopardize your heart health. Magnesium is also important for brain health, detoxification, cellular health and function, energy production, regulation of insulin sensitivity, normal cell division, the optimization of your mitochondria and much more.

Magnesium resides at the center of the chlorophyll molecule, so if you rarely eat fresh leafy greens, you're probably not getting much magnesium from your diet. Furthermore, while eating organic whole foods will help optimize your magnesium intake, it's still not a surefire way to ward off magnesium deficiency, as most soils have become severely depleted of nutrients, including magnesium.

Magnesium absorption is also dependent on having sufficient amounts of selenium, parathyroid hormone and vitamins B6 and D, and is hindered by excess ethanol, salt, coffee and phosphoric acid in soda. Sweating, stress, lack of sleep, excessive menstruation, certain drugs (especially diuretics and proton-pump inhibitors) also deplete your body of magnesium.

For these reasons, many experts recommend taking supplemental magnesium. The recommended dietary allowance for magnesium is 310 to 420 mg per day depending on your age and sex, but many experts believe you may need 600 to 900 mg per day, which is more in line with the magnesium uptake during the Paleolithic period.

Personally, I believe many may benefit from amounts as high as 1 to 2 grams (1,000 to 2,000 mg) of elemental magnesium per day in divided doses, as most have electromagnetic field exposures that simply cannot be mitigated, and the extra magnesium may help lower the damage from that exposure.

The key to effectively using higher doses, however, is to make sure you avoid loose bowels as that will disrupt your gut microbiome, which would be highly counterproductive.

One of the best forms is magnesium threonate, as it appears to be the most efficient at penetrating cell membranes, including your mitochondria and blood-brain barrier. Another effective way to boost your magnesium level is to take Epsom salt (magnesium sulfate) baths, as the magnesium effectively absorbs through your skin.

I prepare a supersaturated solution of Epsom salts by dissolving seven tablespoons of the salt into six ounces of water and heating it until all the salt has dissolved. I pour it into a dropper bottle and then apply it to my skin and rub fresh aloe leaves over it to dissolve it. This is an easy and inexpensive way to increase your magnesium and will allow you to get higher dosages into your body without having to deal with its laxative effects.

Optimizing your magnesium level is particularly important when taking supplemental vitamin D, as your body cannot properly utilize the vitamin if you're your magnesium is insufficient. The reason for this is because magnesium is required for the actual activation of Vitamin D.

If your magnesium level is too low, the vitamin D will simply get stored in its inactive form. As an added boon, when your magnesium level is sufficiently high, it will be far easier to optimize your vitamin D level, as you'll require a far lower dose. In fact, research shows higher magnesium intake helps reduce your risk of vitamin D deficiency — likely by activating more of it.

Homocysteine. Homocysteine is an amino acid in your body and blood obtained primarily from meat consumption. Checking your homocysteine level is a great way to identify a vitamin B6, B9 (folate) and B12 deficiency.

Vitamins B6, B9 and B12 help convert homocysteine into methionine — a building block for proteins. If you don't get enough of these B vitamins, this conversion process is impaired and results in higher homocysteine. Conversely, when you increase intake of B6, B9 and B12, your homocysteine level decreases. Elevated homocysteine is a risk factor for heart disease, and when combined with a low Omega-3 index, it's associated with an increased risk of brain atrophy and dementia.

Vitamins B6, B9 and B12 are also really important for cognition and mental health in general, so identifying and addressing a deficiency in these vitamins can go a long way toward warding off depression and other, even more serious, mental health conditions. If you do take folate and/or B12 it would be best to take the methyl forms of these vitamins.

NMR Lipoprofile. One of the most important tests you can get to determine your heart disease risk is the NMR LipoProfile, which measures your low-density lipoprotein (LDL) particle number. This test also has other markers that can help determine if you have insulin resistance, which is a primary cause of elevated LDL particle number and increased heart disease risk.

Conventional doctors will typically only check your total cholesterol, LDL cholesterol, high-density lipoprotein (HDL) cholesterol and triglycerides. However, these are not very accurate predictors for cardiovascular disease risk, as it's quite possible to have normal total cholesterol and/or normal LDL cholesterol yet have a high LDL particle number.

In a nutshell, it's not the amount of cholesterol that is the main risk factor for heart disease but rather it's the number of cholesterol-carrying LDL particles. The greater the number of LDL particles you have, the more likely it is that you also have oxidized LDL, which tend to be far more atherogenic.

Oxidized LDL is more harmful than normal nonoxidized LDL because it's smaller and denser. This allows it to penetrate the lining of your arteries, where it stimulates plaque formation.

Some groups, such as the National Lipid Association, have started to shift the focus toward LDL particle number instead of total and LDL cholesterol, but it still has not hit mainstream. Fortunately, if you know about it, you can take control of your health and either ask your doctor for this test or order it yourself.

There are several ways to test for your LDL particle number. The NMR Lipoprofile is offered by a lab called Liposcience, and is the test used in most scientific studies on LDL particles. If your LDL particle number is high, chances are you have insulin and leptin resistance, as these are driving causes of high LDL particle numbers.

Endotoxins in your gut will also increase your LDL particle number, and thyroid dysfunction may be at play as well. In the video above, Chris Kresser, an acupuncturist and a licensed integrative medicine clinician, explains how LDL particle number is influenced via these and other mechanisms.

Level 2 Testing

Now, if you have done all this testing and addressed everything and still feel like you have unresolved issues, you need to go to the next level of testing. These days, there are many more tests available to help a practitioner zero in on what is going on. A company called Salveo Diagnostics does very extensive testing in Lipids; Cardiovascular Metabolism, Inflammation and Oxidative Stress; Diabetes/Insulin Resistance, Red Blood Cell Fatty Acid Panel, Hemostasis and Thrombosis, Cholesterol Homeostasis; Gut Health Serum Assessment (Candida); Celiac Disease; Digestion/Absorption/Nutrition/Inflammation; Systemic Auto-immune Conditions; Rheumatoid Arthritis; Thyroid Health Complete Panel (including antibodies); Hormone Health

Assessment; Bone Health Assessment; Electrolytes; Kidney Function; Liver Assessment; Proteins; Iron Studies; and Complete Blood Counts. This is all one test!!

Think of what these results may mean to you. And then they do a companion Gut Health and Stool Assessment. In that, they look at, Intestinal bacteria content; Short Chain Fatty Acids; Gut Inflammation; Digestion/Absorption; Intestinal Permeability; Gastrointestinal Bleeding and Pathogens and that is all from one stool sample. Some insurance companies will pay for this set of tests-some won't. But isn't your health worth it?

Find a Naturopath or an Integrative Doctor that will prescribe these tests for you. Major clinics these days are offering these types of services. Our Inova Clinic System has a Traditional Chinese Medicine Center. Maybe yours does, too.

My wife gave me permission to tell her story. She has been suffering for years from various symptoms that no doctor has been able to resolve, even with all the standardized tests. It was only through the above tests did something significant turn up. As it turns out, she is lacking a key nutrient that helps her use her B vitamins. This is a genetic abnormality. It is huge and can have a major effect on tons of body functions. And, it would have never been found without these more in-depth tests.

At one point in my life, I started losing weight uncontrollably. For months, no doctor could figure it out. I finally went to a naturopath. He ran some tests and decided I had a gluten sensitivity, not Celiac, just sensitivity. He took me off gluten and within one month, my weight fully recovered. Miraculous.

I also recommend a full hormone panel, a hair analysis for heavy metals and mineral balance and a urine mold test. The mold test is expensive but can save your life if you are having serious mold-related issues or other unexplained issues like headaches, fatigue, unreasonable obesity, depression, brain fog.

Level 3 Testing

There are many other genetic tests, much more detailed than the above these days. DNA fit can tell you what you should be eating and avoiding to optimize your health. 23 and Me can help you Identify your abnormalities, then you can send those results off to an expert like Ben Lynch and have his software tell exactly what to concentrate on to improve your health. Some people do this just for prevention, even if you are feeling great, just to make sure you are on the right track and know what your genetics are telling you. A company called Viome does a very detailed stool analysis based on a technology they bought from NASA, where they analyze genetic material rather than look for specific species of pathogens.

Keep in mind however, it is not your genes that determine your health, it is whether they are expressed that determines your health, and optimal expression is under your control through your beliefs, diet and lifestyle choices. This is called Epigenetics, as discussed in the chapters above.

CHAPTER 18

Macro and Micro Nutrients

It is critical that we all understand the basic needs of the human body. Now more than ever. Why? Because we can no longer depend on the soil or even perhaps the seas to provide the nutrition we need, either from plants or from meat. The soils have become depleted. Even though they can grow plants, the plants are unhealthy, needing chemicals to stay alive and defend against predators, and needing fertilizers that only contain just the bare essentials to keep the plant growing, which in turn feed livestock and humans.

We must keep in mind, without the plants we all die, even if all we ever eat is meat. Humans are like that too. Just getting the bare essentials will get us only to a certain point in our lives before our vital driving life force gives out at a premature age. Then disease sets in. And we enter our unhealthy stage, wondering why we are sick and in pain. So, as Dr. Furhman says, become a nutrivore. Go for the highest density most nutritious foods on the planet. These days, that takes effort.

Most people think in terms of the macros: Proteins, Carbs and Fats and totally miss the micros: Vitamins, Minerals and phyto (plant) nutrients. The macros will keep you alive for a time, but not healthy. Eventually, your body will be starving for the micros and you enter a disease state. In fact, excessive macros, like fat and sugar, can fool you into a false state of satiation, while your cells are starving for micros. Your body sends signals…I need more micros…feed me, but it does not know how to say micros, just that it is hungry. So, you eat more sugar and fat and still don't feed your cells' functions, just produce more empty calories, devoid of what it takes to keep your cells humming smoothly.

So, you keep eating more empty calories and still get that unfulfilled feeling, causing obesity while at the same time are in a severe state of malnutrition. Then you are stuck with a double whammy: inflammation and tons of problems caused by obesity and starvation due to malnutrition of the cells.

What are these micros and how do we get them? If you go keto, or Atkins or any other popular diet, if you do not include your micros, you will eventually damage yourself. Further, if you are really keyed in on micros and do your best to cover the micros with your food choices and say, superfood powders, it may be possible to avoid supplements.

But that takes way more effort than most people want to expend, or more money than they are willing to invest in their health. So, the alternative, is to invest in high quality supplements to get the micros you need. And further, these days, I am not sure there is any way to get all the micros you need, simply from whole foods, due to soil depletion. So as insurance, even if you are very diligent, careful and thoughtful about the food you eat, it would be worthwhile to add supplements to your dietary plan.

Given the above and without going into the benefits of each, here are some generalized supplements I would recommend as a minimum for 5 days a week. I would not take anything 7 days a week.

You need to give your body a nutritional rest to avoid allergies and other conditions of over use.

Magnesium: start small with an eighth of a teaspoon of miracle magnesium in a cup of boiling water, then build to higher levels.

MSM: great for Sulphur. Two teaspoons a day as a minimum.

Iodine: 4 drops a day if you do not consume seaweed consistently

Fulvic Minerals: Energy boost 70, one capful a day

High Quality Food-Based Multi-vitamin/mineral pill

Polyphenols: I use Dr. Gundry's Vital Reds, one scoop daily

Vitamin D3/K2: Designs for Health, 1 pill a day (keep your D3 blood levels above 50)

Vitamin B complex: Pure brand, liquid B complex, sub lingual (squirt a dropper full under your tongue and hold it there for few minutes.

Fiber: Fresh ground flax seed, 1 tablespoon,

Omega 3/6: Two krill oil pills, one Borage oil

CHAPTER 19

Herbs, Spices and Essential Oils

Make sure and include in your normal diet a plentiful supply of miraculous herbs and spices. They have incredible healing powers that science has proven over and over and over again. I cannot emphasize their abilities to help you prevent disease and stay healthy. Just look at the one, the mighty, the towering orange colored spice of Turmeric.

Some of the most amazing demonstrated properties include:

Destroying Multi-Drug Resistant Cancer

Destroying Cancer Stem Cells (arguably, the root of all cancer)

Protecting Against Radiation-Induced Damage

Reducing Unhealthy Levels of Inflammation

Protecting Against Heavy Metal Toxicity

Preventing and Reversing Alzheimer's Disease Associated Pathologies

Who would not want this? It is almost as if we were designed to consume this spice and other plant compounds as a normal part of staying healthy on this earth, and the further we drift away from natural foods into processed foods, the more we stray from our original design for longevity on the planet. And this is only a few properties of turmeric. A GrennMedinfo search of medical literature on turmeric revealed over **580** health benefits, and/or its primary polyphenol known as curcumin. Turmeric has compounds that curcumin does not. That is why I consume both turmeric and curcumin around five days a week, turmeric powder and curcumin/cayenne pills. Granted, turmeric is strong tasting, so I mix it in with everything I can think of: my morning breakfast formula, my salads, my smoothies, anything to hide the taste. And, some people actually like it. Go figure.

I could go on and on. Garlic is a fantastic antibiotic as well as ginger. Cinnamon helps control blood sugar. Stevia, the artificial sweetener, has been shown to be effective against Lyme disease. Essential oils are excellent antimicrobials and have helped many with aroma therapy. Inhaling them can help kill sinus infections and ingesting them can kill unwanted digestive pathogens. They are also effective in fighting cancer. I could write a whole book on them and many people have. I recommend this book: *The Healing Power of Essential Oils: Soothe Inflammation, Boost Mood, Prevent Autoimmunity, and Feel* Paperback – March 13, 2018 by Eric Zielinski D.C. (Author)

There is no end to these powerful healing compounds so it would be wise start including a good supply in your regular lifestyle habits.

CHAPTER 20

The Healing Powers

Love, Spirituality, Prayer, Meditation, Forgiveness, Gratitude and the Placebo Effect (Are they related?)

The mind body connection is a well-recognized part of medical science. As professor Jason M. Satterfield teaches in his course, "Mind-Body Medicine: The New Science of Optimal Health," there are many physiological pathways between thoughts, feelings and emotions and the function of the human body. In his course, he talks about the autonomic nervous system and the difference in effects between the parasympathetic (rest, heal and digest) and the sympathetic (fight or flight) on the human body. The mental state you are in puts you either in the parasympathetic mode or sympathetic mode.

He talks about the Hypothalamus-Pituitary-Adrenal (HPA) brain-body connection effecting our vital hormone production (cortisol dysregulation from adrenal HPA problems due to excess stress can ruin your life). He talks about the emotional effect on weakening the Immune system (In fact, there is a whole new branch of science called Pschoneuroimmunology that studies the effect of psychology on the immune system, and the effect it is huge)!! He talks about our genes and the possibility that our behavior effects genetic expression through altering our epigenetic tags. He talks about the effects of personality on health. This just a sample of potential links between the body and the mind.

Countless studies on testing the effectiveness of drugs have shown that the placebo effect is real, meaning, the mere thought that taking a curative agent, even though it might be a sugar pill, can have the same exact effect or better than taking the actual drug. Instead of demonizing the placebo effect, we need to harness, nurture and make use of this tremendous healing power. And the "nocebo" effect is real as well, meaning, being told you have a terminal disease could kill you way before the actual disease does. Bruce Lipton in his famous book, "The Biology of Belief," showed belief can affect biological function at the cellular level. This is incredible!

If you experience Love in your life, love yourself and are connected to a constant source of non-judgmental love, would that not create a since of bliss and relaxation and stress lowering throughout your entire nervous system? Would that not help your immune system and your hormonal system? If you are a spiritual person, you could feel that love coming from the divine in a prayer. Wouldn't that be a similar state as a meditative state, where you block out the world around you, if even for a few minutes, moving you into the parasympathetic mode (rest, heal and digest), allowing your body to rebuild and heal?

If you repeat affirmations of positive healing thoughts, is that not like a placebo, recognizing the placebo effect is real? Those positive thoughts, if repeated often, should soak in and become real, just as your belief that you are taking the real drug, when in fact, you are taking the sugar pill. In the world of mind-body effects, this has tremendous healing potential.

Forgiveness and gratitude are very special healing forces for your body. It puts you in a completely different mindset, and by now, you know there are many connections between the mind and body. But these two healing forces are easier said than practiced. People endure great hardship in their lives, through parental abuse and addictions, through workplace abuse, through bullying, through friendship abuse, through perceived failures, self-judgment…all leading to pent up anger, frustration, regrets, guilt and emotional pain that can last a lifetime and hold you in the grip of an unhealthy body.

It is very hard to move into a state of forgiveness and gratitude when all you feel is anger and disappointment, right? So how does one do this? Well, one way is to reverse the normal progression of life here on earth. Normally, feelings lead to emotions which lead to thoughts, which lead to actions and then words. If the feelings and emotions are not there, then try reversing the order. Use the words and repeat words every day; that is what affirmations are all about. Send out to the universe what you want to feel and do it often. Post it on your mirror and on your door posts. Say it when you rise up and when you lay down, "I forgive you for _____. I forgive myself for ______. I will no longer hurt myself by holding on to this anger. I am grateful for _____ and for ________. I give to God my burdens so that I can heal and be who I was meant to be. Keep saying this or thinking it as you lay in bed before you get up and before you go to sleep, whether you feel it or not. See if over time you can "feel" it. Demonstrate gratitude to others, act on it. Demonstrate forgiveness. Words and actions first, then hopefully thoughts, emotions and feelings will naturally follow. It is worth try is it not? Break the chains of the bondage you have been under. Your body will thank you for it.

Here is a piece from Alberto Villodo, PhD; on Gratitude:

There is a magical moment in the ritual of Thanksgiving when we express appreciation for our blessings. Embracing gratefulness — allowing the sensation of gratitude to wash over us — can induce feelings of calm, love, warmth, happiness, stability and splendor. It changes who we are. The practice of gratitude converts to a cellular, physiological, biochemical, and neurological experience. Exercised on a regular basis, gratitude has a positive impact on our emotions, personality, physical health, career, and social life.

Gratitude brings harmony to the countless cells and microorganisms that make up our body and function in exquisite synchronicity to maintain our health. It leads to grace – the grace that enables us to take on the stewardship of all that surrounds us. It opens our eyes and helps us see the beauty present everywhere, in every moment and circumstance. The shamanic traditions of the ancient Earthkeepers – the aboriginal societies of this world – were founded on the practice of immense gratitude. It permeated their lives and fueled their daily activities. It linked them to the Ancient Ones, to Mother Earth, Father Sun, Grandmother Moon, to the vast Cosmos, and above all the Great Spirit. Gratitude allowed them to see beauty as they toiled, survived, and evolved. The world will always mirror back to us what we are at any given moment. If we are immersed in gratitude, beauty, and peace, our world will reflect that. This is how we dream a new and better world into being.

But how do we express gratitude when we feel awful, when we are in pain, anger, or despair? We bring our hands together, bow our heads, and address whatever it is that we identify as the Source, saying "Thank you for this moment .. for this breath ... for this beating heart..." We *find something* to be thankful for—a loyal pet, a kind friend, a drop of water. The moment you find something to be thankful for, a blotch of color begins to take over the landscape. Don't make your practice of thankfulness dependent on your mood – when you *feel* like giving thanks. Do it when times are tough. It may take a while to cultivate; there is a reason it is called a "practice."

Gratitude, the feeling that we're blessed, helps us to stop being enslaved to our to-do lists and remember why we came here: To love, to learn, to grow, to discover what we can do to participate in the unfolding work of art called creation. It also reminds us of what we most value, and inspires us to stop procrastinating, awaken from the nightmare of frenetic but meaningless activity, and start truly living the way we want to live, with boldness and originality.

In Munay,

Alberto Villoldo, PhD

Perhaps all we do when we meditate or pray is open ourselves up to the healing love of the universe, lowering our stress levels and allowing our body to function more in parasympathetic mode, as it was designed. Perhaps eating natural food is a way of ingesting love through the selections we make, if that food is a result of a loving power that gives us sunlight, that grows our plants to provide us sustenance during our time here on earth.

There is much we do not know still about the mind body connection and how our cells stay in constant communication with each other through chemical signaling pathways and light emissions. We know our cells emit light, and we know the speed of light is very, very fast, so our mind and body may be working together more closely than we could possibly imagine.

There are some cancer treatment centers in the world that use light as a therapy, claiming that cancer cells are dark and devoid of light. Since sunlight is in a sense captured in the plants we eat, food then becomes the mechanism of transfer, a transfer of sunlight deep into our tissues through the consumption of fresh, whole, organic raw foods. The entire field of light at the cellular level is very exciting and new. I cannot wait to see more results of scientific study in this area.

As science progresses, we will learn more and more in this area so my advice is to use what we know already and do everything you can to bring more balance back into your life, keeping stress to a minimum and staying in parasympathetic mode as much as possible in this hectic life we lead.

The whole universe is in balance. Look at how a galaxy forms. It starts with a massive black hole in stellar gasses. The gravity of the high mass center of the black hole pulls in the matter of the gasses, ever increasing the mass of the center while at the same time stars are forming in the interstellar gasses surrounding the black whole. The black whole acts as a drain in your sink. Just as water forms a vortex as it is pulled down the drain, so do all the gasses and suns start to swirl in a vortex surrounding the black hole drain, pulling in all matter around it. Left without balance, the entire forming galaxy would be sucked into the black hole, never to be seen again.

But something strange happens. Instead of growing infinitely more massive, the black hole reaches a tipping point at which time it cannot accept any more mass from the stellar gasses and shoots them out into space in huge gas/matter rays, thus turning into Quasars that we can see through our telescopes. Eventually, it reaches a balance or equilibrium. No more gasses are shot out into space. Everything settles down and a more mature galaxy is born, where the stars swirl in a vortex, pulled towards the center of the massive black whole but are not consumed.

Thus, our Milky Way becomes livable, through balance and homeostasis. Our bodies are a reflection of this balance. And when we get out of balance, our bodies will do everything in its power to restore this balance (see Laws of Life #16), in thousands of interconnected physiological and emotional systems we are just beginning to understand.

CHAPTER 21

Detoxing in a Toxic World

Chemical and Heavy Metal Detoxing. Detox, detox, detox. I have mentioned this before but not brought it out as a separate chapter. It is critically important, due to several of the dots, especially since there is no way to avoid chemical and toxin exposure in today's world. If you are healthy, all you need is maintenance levels of detoxing. If you are sick, then you need increased frequency of detoxing. I detox at several levels. Once a month, I do two rounds of coffee enemas, then follow that with a water enema.

In the winter months, I get in my infrared sauna once a week for some good sweating, followed by a cold shower for my cryo therapy. Once a year, I do a citrus/oil flush. And then once a year, I do a Cytodetox with Binder (a charcoal product, both are available from Dr. Pompa). That seems to keep me at a fairly good level. But if I am feeling sluggish, I can always step it up with whatever I need. I also do intermittent fasting every other day, skipping breakfast and instead have Brain Octane and coconut oil in my non-caffeinated hot drink in the morning during my fasting days.

I also brew up some of DocofDetox daily detox tea and add in Pau De Arco (from Starwest Botanicals) to the mixture. Then

I place in the fridge (makes a gallon of tea) and pour the tea in my morning breakfast bowl Monday, Wednesday and Friday.

Mis-folded Protein Detoxing. There are many reasons why the body folds proteins incorrectly, everything from something called glycation, where too much sugar consumption causes it to attach to protein creating Advanced Glycation Endproducts (AGE), to too much of a certain kind of Reactive Oxygen Species or oxidants that effect protein folding, to things and reasons we have no clue about. Either way, the message is:

Mis-folded proteins do not work, build up in the system (or brain) and need to be fixed or eliminated from our body. As it turns out, our body has a natural way to do this called autophagy. We just have to be aware of it and create the circumstances for it to do internal house cleaning through fasting and/or vigorous exercise. Yes, fasting creates the conditions for our body to enter autophagy. In a recent article from Harvard Medical School communication dates February 21, 2019, I quote:

"The body's ability to adapt to changing conditions and shifting physiologic demands is essential to its survival. To ensure cellular performance and the health of the entire organism, each cell must be able to dispose of damaged or unnecessary proteins. Now, a study from the Blavatnik Institute at Harvard Medical School (HMS) shows that intense exercise, fasting, and an array of hormones can activate cells' built-in protein-disposal systems and enhance their ability to purge defective, toxic, or unneeded proteins.

The findings, published February 2019 in PNAS, reveal a previously unknown mechanism that is triggered by fluctuations in hormone levels, which signal changes in physiologic conditions.

"Our findings show that the body has a built-in mechanism for cranking up the molecular machinery responsible for waste-protein removal that is so critical for the cells' ability to adapt to new conditions," said Alfred Goldberg, senior author on the study and professor of cell biology at the Blavatnik Institute.

Malfunctions in the cells' protein-disposal machinery can lead to the accumulation of misfolded proteins, which clog up the cell, interfere with its functions, and, over time, precipitate the development of diseases, including neurodegenerative conditions such as amyotrophic lateral sclerosis and Alzheimer's."

So, I encourage everyone to do your research, and get into some form of regular fasting with something called Intermittent Fasting, or by slowly working your way into one day water fasting. Check out Mike Mutzel at High Intensity Health if you want to learn more about metabolic detoxing and autophagy.

I know this is a huge change for some of us, but I guarantee you will feel better over time with consistent detoxing.

CHAPTER 22

My Morning Rituals

This is not a static thing nor should it be. We have to adjust for our own bodies and our bodies change over time, so we have to change with them. Many people could not handle the portions I use because they are not used to such a massive dose of healthy items. When you give this a try, go easy. Start slow. And build up to these levels over time.

I try to keep my body off guard, so I vary my routine every other day.

MONDAY, WEDNESDAY, FRIDAY

First thing in the morning: Full body vibration on my vibrating plate for 15 minutes. Then, hot water with dissolved magnesium (one half a teaspoon), and MSM (one teaspoon), 4 drops iodine, one half squeezed lemon juice and a little local raw honey with a couple shakes of cayenne pepper. Use this to down my first set of pills: a probiotic (SBO from Dr. Axe), Mega Green

Tea Extract from LifeExtension, 2 Beta Glucans from Transfer Point.

Then I get ready for work and come back and prepare my breakfast bowl: Start with Vital Reds (from Dr. Gundry), add heaping spoonful of Immortal Machine from David Wolfe, a scoop of Protein Powder from David Wolfe, a heaping spoonful of collagen (Dr. Axe), heaping spoonful of organic moringa, heaping spoonful of Tonic Alchemy (Dragon Herbs), organic Goat Colostrum (one day a week), a few shakes of turmeric powder, a spoonful of fresh organic ground peanut butter, three spoonfuls of raw organic hemp seed, half spoonful of Apple Peel Powder (Apple Boost), one spoonful of dehydrated lemon peel powder (make it myself), one spoonful of fresh ground flax seed, then organic wild blueberries and strawberries, a good squirt of filtered organic flax oil.

Then I add a premade detox tea (from DocofDetox Daily tea, plus Pau-de-arco). Stir that all up and eat it for breakfast.
After that, I down more pills: one D3/K Ultra 10K (from Designs for Health), one curcumin from DocofDetox, one Eye Protector (from pure synergy), one Tongkat Ali (from Health Solution for increased Testosterone), two Krill Oil (from Dr. Mercola) and one Borage Oil. Then, before I get in the car, I put sublingual B complex and vitamin D3 (from Pure) under my tongue for about 10 minutes as I drive in to work.

TUESDAY, THURSDAY, SATURDAY

Intermittent Fasting days, so I start with hot water, dissolve magnesium and MSM, with four drops iodine, then add raw organic ground up cacao nibs. Then add one spoonful of coconut oil and one spoonful of Brain Octane (from Asprey) along with stevia, and one Daily Advantage from Dave Asprey in my drink.

Then head off for work. At work, I have a good workout in the gym on Tuesday and Thursday, my 16 hour fasting days. It is great to work out during fasting periods, putting you into fat burning quicker and also into internal house cleaning quicker. I have started experimenting with a Metabolic Monday. On Mondays, I have been doing a 24-hour water fast. The more I do it, the easier it gets. It is kind of weird emotionally, but once I got over that, I really do not get hungry during the fast. Very interesting. Guess I am becoming more fat-adapted, able to equally burn sugar or fat for fuel, and feeling good that I am clearing old junk proteins from my cells. If I do a water fast Monday, then I don't fast again until Thursday.

These are my current morning rituals. If something else is working for you, please send me your morning regimens so I can share with others. If you'd like help creating your own morning ritual, please contact me.

CHAPTER 23

Body Weight Management

The Emerging Truth

No matter what doctors may tell you about weight loss, we now know that it is not a simple, calories in/calories out solution for most of us (but for some, it is!). In the toxic physical, electrical and emotional world we live in, there could be many factors forcing your body to retain fat, making it near impossible to get to your desired weight or get off a plateau you may be stuck in. This is going to be one of those fire hose lessons where I will try and cover as many factors as possible in the space allotted, while keeping it out of the deep biochemical weeds. Much of this information comes from a great PhD researcher by the name of Stephan Guyenet who released a book called, *The Hungry Brain*.

This is about the physiology of body weight. I highly recommend it. Also, the great Dr. Hyman, who has exposed and shared some of the greatest lipid (fat) researchers and scientists to the general public, so he knows what he is talking about. But as always, I have included many other sources and added my perspectives and information when it is appropriate. My overall message is this: everyone is different, and no single diet works for everyone. Fad diets usually do not work for the long haul. But, in order to figure out what works best for you and your weight loss program, you have to do something, try something, change your routine, make observations, become your own practitioner, record your average (not daily but weekly) progress, make adjustments, see what works.

So, let's dive in.

First off, your body does talk in calories, it talks in neurotransmitters and hormones. The concept of calories is nothing more than a physics term to denote the amount of heat produced. In the nutritional world, they burn different food types and see how much heat it produces. That gives us a rough idea of the calorie content of each food but has no meaning to our physiology. We do burn fuel and by now you know that there are only two fuels for us, glucose and fat. And supposedly glucose produces less energy than the same weight of fat, about half.

But anyways, your body's weight management system and balancing system hinges on hormones and neurotransmitters, not calories. There is a pleasure center/satiation center in the hypothalamus called the nucleus accumbens and our brain is hard wired to respond to certain foods, namely: sugar, fat, salt, protein and glutamate, not vitamins or minerals. So those are the foods that are going to cause dopamine production and the satiation feeling. Now, on the hormone side, your fat cells produce a hormone called Leptin and the more Leptin you have, the less hungry you will be.

This is a control mechanism to keep your body fat at a certain level, thus acting as your fat thermostat like your home thermostat. If you are coming from an obese state to a slim state, it can be very difficult to lose and keep off the weight, because your body is defending the set point on the thermostat. Coupled with that, just like drug addictions where you need more and more to achieve the same effect, with more and more fat producing more and more leptin, your brain develops leptin resistance, keeping your body thinking that you are in a state of starvation, making you turn to your satiating foods to get satisfied, thus adding even more fat to your body.

Of course, there is genetic variability involved so everyone reacts differently to differing levels of leptin. But in general, these are the basic body fat controls in your system. Other hormones also enter the equation. Cortisol, your stress hormone, also increases Leptin resistance, so the more stress you are under, the hungrier you will be. Insulin also controls sugar levels in the blood and sugar storage in fat cells. Thyroid hormones control how quickly we burn off our fuel sources. So as usual, we are system of systems and each of these pieces are discussed below. But, one way to reset Leptin sensitivity is to eat a simple whole foods diet, no processed foods, no refined sugars.

Time after time we have seen slender native populations adopt an industrial diet and become obese because of it. Food scientists understand this stuff and use this information to purify and extract the very substances (sugar, salt, fat and glutamate) that stimulate our pleasure centers to sell their product. This purified extract eventually causes; increased fat stores, Leptin resistance, starvation syndrome, more eating and thus bigger profits. Brilliant!! But it is killing us. You can also use increased grass-fed protein as a satiator if you need it, to help you get off all other refined and processed foods.

So, with that introduction, there is actually more to the story… here are the things to pay attention to when trying to lose and maintain a healthy body weight:

Nutritional Imbalances: Over 30 percent of American diets fall short in nutrients like magnesium, iodine and Vitamins C, D3, E, and A. Over 80 percent of Americans have low Vitamin D levels. Nine out of 10 people are deficient in Omega-3 fatty acids which, among other things, help cool inflammation and control blood sugar levels. Sugar is a double whammy, it spikes insulin causing fat retention and insulin resistance, plus, it is empty of micro nutrients, causing vast nutritional deficiencies. You must, must, must have the right nutrition to power your mitochondria.

Your mitochondria burn calories and therefore keep your body weight under control. Reduced mitochondrial function and numbers/density = increased body fat. Much of the processed foods today are a nutritional waist land. Even the organic foods can come from nutritionally deficient soils. These days I have finally broken down and recommend a multi-vitamin/mineral supplement for everyone. There are many good products on the market. Key things to look for are no fillers, no GMOs, no oils and a good variety of up to 70 different minerals. Don't skimp on the cost because lower cost usually means lower doses and poorer quality. Some, you are simply throwing your money away. But shifting away from sugar to whole foods will take you a long way to better nutrient density.

Look at Dr. Fuhrman's food density ratings, that will give you a clue as to the highest most nutrient dense foods. And your vitamins and minerals do not have to come in the same package. You can take a multi-vitamin as a pill and take a mineral supplement as a liquid. I always try to keep synthetics to a minimum, so I lean towards a whole food plant based multi-vitamin and mineral products. Those are usually packed with other great foods for you such as green superfoods, enzymes, polyphenols and probiotics.

Gut Microbiome Imbalances: From both animal and human models, we know that the bacteria in our gut can have profound effects on weight and metabolism, through many types of mechanisms. Some bacteria extract more energy from food, leading to weight gain, while other bacteria will extract less energy from your food, leading to weight loss. Studies have shown that taking the gut bacteria from a thin mouse and putting it into a fat mouse can cause the fat mouse to lose dramatic amounts of weight without changing its diet. Some bacteria trigger inflammation leading to a leaky gut, while others are anti-inflammatory. Inflammation triggers insulin resistance and diabetes, independent of your caloric intake. So, clearly, it's important to heal your gut if it is damaged by imbalances.

I typically recommend working with a Functional Medicine practitioner/ holistic health coach, but there are many things you can do on your own to cultivate a healthy microbiome and heal a leaky gut. The best policy is to eat fermented food daily or take a large variety/volume probiotic or both (like me!) and consume grass-fed bone broth as much as possible, without becoming constipated. Another piece to the gut equation is prebiotics, not probiotics. Prebiotics are foods that feed your probiotics. We are talking about certain starches that are tough for you to digest but are excellent for your good bacteria.

Fiber and Resistant starches fall into this category, plus others. Google prebiotics and start fitting them into your routine.

Now, here is an interesting paradox.

Most your bacteria live and populate in the lower large intestine. But, you may have an upper small intestine infection called SIBO or Small Intestine Bacterial Overgrowth. In this case, the very prebiotic fiber and perhaps probiotic that may be good for you, can cause you terrible gas and bloating and pain. If this is the case, you need a whole different strategy to rid yourself of this upper intestinal infection before you can go on healing your gut with normal protocols. You would be surprised how many people actually have SIBO and all sorts of problems that it can cause. You can test for SIBO, but I have had very good results administering Allicin (a Garlic extract) and or Berberine to clear up SIBO. Start with Allicin for at least a month as see if you feel better, then try Berberine if you are not seeing improvement. You must get this cleared before you can go on to improve your gut health in other ways.

You may need several natural antibiotics to tame the bad bacteria in your system like colloidal silver, but there are many others. Here are some other things you can do for gut health/microbiome diversity:

- **Eat whole, unprocessed, unrefined foods.** One of the best ways to maintain gut health involves cutting out the sugar and refined carbs and jacking up gut-supporting fiber. Seventy-five percent of your plate should be vegetables and plant-based foods. Your gut bugs really love these high-fiber plant foods.
- **Eat good fats and get an oil change.** The good fats we mentioned earlier (like Omega-3 fats and monounsaturated fats, such as unheated extra-virgin olive oil) will help with decreasing inflammation, giving healthy gut bugs a chance to flourish.
- **Supplement smartly.** Studies find Omega-3 fatty acids can support healthy gut flora, aside from their other numerous benefits, like reducing inflammation. If you're not regularly eating wild-caught fatty fish, you should definitely supplement with an essential fatty acid formula. Take a strong probiotic supplement as well. This helps reduce gut inflammation while cultivating health and the growth of good bacteria. I like Dr. Axe's SBO probiotic, especially if you are not used to a lot of fermented food.
- **Add more coconut oil.** Studies demonstrate anti-inflammatory and weight loss benefits from adding Medium Chain Triglyceride or MCT oils. Some of my favorite fats, coconut oil and coconut butter, contains these fabulous fat-burning MCTs.

- **Remove inflammatory fats.** Cut out bad, inflammatory Omega-6 rich fats like vegetable oils. Replace these with healthier oils like extra-virgin olive oil and coconut oil.
- **Add fiber-rich foods**. Nuts, seeds, and a special fiber called glucomannan provide prebiotics and feed our healthy bacteria. Also, whole Chia seed or freshly ground flax seeds are excellent high fiber additions to your diet.
- **Add fermented foods.** Sauerkraut, kimchi, organic tempeh, and miso contain good amounts of probiotics so your healthy gut bugs can be fruitful and multiply. Other sources are kombucha (a fermented tea), low-sugar yogurt and well-aged cheese (if dairy does not bother you). You can also buy fermented veggies in your grocery store to add to all your salads. Most of them taste very good. Or, of course you can make them at home. There are multiple free videos on line to teach you how to do this.
- **Inflammation and immune function:** Science now clearly identifies chronic disease and aging as a state of inflammation. And it's not just allergies, asthma, arthritis, or autoimmunity that are the causes of inflammation. We now know that diabetes and obesity are inflammatory problems, as are heart disease, cancer, depression, autism, and dementia.

  Your fat cells produce inflammatory molecules that perpetuate weight gain and disease. Other factors can trigger weight-gain inducing inflammation, independent of caloric intake. There are many other triggers for inflammation that also promote weight gain – including: infections (such as viruses), mold toxins, environmental toxins, food allergens (such as gluten and dairy), a poor-quality processed diet that is high in sugar and Omega-6 refined oils, and low in fiber.

All of these trigger inflammations, which then creates insulin resistance and promotes weight gain. *The Blood Sugar Solution* and *Eat Fat, Get Thin* by Dr. Hyman are designed to be powerful anti-inflammatory programs. Take a look at my chapter, *Inflammation and What to Do About It*. Learning to identify the various hidden sources of inflammation is often critical for those who are stuck in the vicious cycle of the dreaded plateau. We also know that inflammation is at the root of many diseases, so it is worth lowering even if you weight is under control. You can get a basic measure of your body's inflammatory state by measuring your blood C Reactive Protein levels. Just ask your doc to do this, he will know what it is. You are looking for results of under 1.0.

- **Environmental toxins:** Many doctors look down on the whole idea of detoxification. But if you were to ask them what happens when your kidneys or liver fail, or if you're constipated for weeks on end, you'd quickly find out just how important the detoxification process really is. Detoxification is a natural process that occurs all the time in the body, though our personal ability to detoxify can become hindered for a variety of reasons.

  Unfortunately, in our modern world, we are exposed to a huge burden of toxins from our environment and our diet. There are many ways to detoxify your body and is worthy of a complete chapter (see my chapter on Detox). I also give you some ideas below. I use a combination of an herbal tea five days a week, a coffee enema once a month and a liver/gall bladder flush annually along with a heavy metal remover/charcoal treatment once a year.

  These toxins, including plastics, pesticides, phthalates, bisphenol A, flame retardants, metals like mercury, lead, arsenic – and any one of the 80,000 chemicals introduced into our world since the industrial revolution – have been shown to interfere with metabolism and cause weight gain even in the absence of extra calories. These environmental toxins are called obesogens.

There are many mechanisms by which toxins promote weight gain – affecting your metabolism, your hormones, and your brain function. Reducing your exposure to environmental toxins is entirely possible. There is a lot you can do to cut your exposure to toxins and help your body eliminate the ones it may already contain.

Eat organic when you can and follow the Environmental Working Group's list of the "Dirty Dozen and Clean Fifteen." This list helps identify the fruits and vegetables that are more or less likely to contain agricultural chemical residues.

Stop eating mercury. Avoid big fish with lots of mercury – such as large fish tuna and swordfish.

Eat clean, organic animal products by choosing grass-fed or pasture-raised animals that haven't been exposed to hormones or antibiotics. These responsibly raised products cost more, but the reduced exposure to these additives and toxins is well worth the cost.

Be sure to filter your water. Use a carbon or reverse osmosis filter to get rid of hidden contaminants in your water supply. Drink 6 ounces of fresh filtered water every hour up until about 6 PM. Then stop hydrating so you can get a good night's rest. Please see my chapter on Hydration for more fascinating information about the latest science on water. It will surprise you.

Eating lots of fiber helps you poop at least once a day – this a very important part of the detoxification process!

Add 1 to 2 cups of cruciferous vegetables daily to assist with detoxification. This includes foods like broccoli, kale, and bok choy, and lots of garlic, onions, ginger, and turmeric.

Don't forget to sweat – this is the body's natural mechanism to excrete toxins – so I recommend getting outside to play or participating in your favorite exercise – or go relax in a sauna! Sunlighten makes wonderful home saunas. I have a half moon floor model called "Solo". You lay down and slide it up over you and it is very easy to store and uses a normal 110 outlet.

Take supplements that support detoxification including selenium, zinc, Vitamin C, and a Vitamin B-Complex.

Take special glutathione boosting compounds such as n-acetyl-cysteine, alpha lipoic acid, and milk thistle, which also support your liver.

Be careful about what you put on your body; your hair products, make-up, deodorants, suntan lotion can all carry toxins into your body through your skin.

Look into chelation therapies, compounds that bind to heavy metals and pull them out of your system. Every year, once a year, I run through a chelation protocol with two bottles of CytoDetox with compound called BIND, a charcoal-based compound. You can get BIND on Dr. Pompa's website but will have to work through a chiropractor or other licensed practitioner to get CytoDetox (names should be available through Dr. Pompa's website, or you can contact me at bob@conscioushealthclub.com. Plus, during the winter time, I get under my infrared sauna once a week for a good sweat for 20 minutes or so. This is an excellent way to reduce heavy metals from your body.

Troubles with Metabolism

There are many things that affect the number and function of your mitochondria, and therefore your metabolism, that you can control. The greatest damage to our energy system comes from our diet. When we eat lots of sugary, processed, inflammatory foods like refined oils, or we simply consume too much food, we overload our energy factories and they become damaged.

Environmental toxins like pesticides and mercury, along with hidden infections and stress, also harm our energy systems. Even your gut microbiome can be a problem if the unhealthy inflammatory bugs outweigh the good bugs. Essentially, anything that causes inflammation (also known as oxidative stress) damages the mitochondria.

The natural act of aging and most chronic diseases– including obesity, diabetes, heart disease, and dementia – are related to mitochondrial dysfunction.

To boost your mitochondria and fire up your metabolism, I recommend eating real, whole foods, avoiding flour, moving more often and faster, reducing toxic exposure, keeping a healthy gut, and taking energy boosting nutrients. Here are my top supplements for boosting mitochondria: Acetyl-L-carnitine, Alpha-lipoic acid, Coenzyme Q10, N-acetyl-cysteine, NADH, D-ribose, Resveratrol. Also, you can help clear toxins from your cells by intermittent fasting.

Do this by skipping your breakfast meal and starting your calorie intake around Noon to 2:00 pm. You can do this twice a week and see how you feel. It takes a while to get used to it. You can help your fast by consuming some decaf coffee in the morning and adding some coconut oil or MCT oil in your coffee. That should help you skip your morning meal without getting hungry until 1:00 or 2:00 pm. Drink lots of water!

Furthermore, your mitochondria are surrounded by a protective barrier wall, much like your cell wall; meaning, mainly composed of fats. Eliminating bad fats from your diet will go a long way to making your energy factories healthy.

Hormonal Imbalances/Autonomic Nervous System

The hormone that has the greatest connection to weight gain and disease is insulin – specifically too much of it. *Eat Fat Get Thin*, is all about how to naturally regulate insulin to shift from fat storage to fat burning.

There are other hormones that are dynamically interacting every minute, which also affects your weight and health. The hormones most likely to affect your weight are thyroid, cortisol, and sex hormones.

Thyroid

Research shows hypothyroidism, or low-thyroid function, affects one in five women and one in ten men. Unfortunately, in over half of these cases, this condition isn't diagnosed.

Many things contribute to these imbalances. *The Ultra Thyroid Solution*, explains how diet, nutrient deficiencies, stress, and environmental toxins impact your thyroid and how to address these problems.

A common cause of hypothyroidism is gluten intolerance.

Other major culprits that interfere with thyroid function include pesticides and heavy metals. Nutrient deficiencies can also slow things down. Your thyroid needs specific nutrients to run optimally including selenium, zinc, iodine, and Omega-3 fats.

Most doctors don't test for thyroid function correctly. Even when they do diagnose it, they don't treat it effectively by optimizing thyroid function through diet, supplements, and the right thyroid hormone replacement therapy.

That's unfortunate since thyroid function plays a vital role in maintaining a healthy weight and hypothyroidism is a major player in weight-loss resistance. Dr. Hyman has found these four strategies can optimize thyroid function and weight loss:

Get the right tests. Ask your doctor to check your thyroid stimulating hormone (TSH and free T3 and T4, as well as thyroid antibodies including thyroid peroxidase (TPO) and anti-thyroglobulin antibodies (TGAb).

Some people may need to dig deeper and get a special test called reverse T3 to learn if something like heavy metals (mercury), pesticides, yeast, or nutritional deficiencies like selenium, vitamin D, zinc, or even iodine could block thyroid hormone function. Reverse T3 is the brake that stops your thyroid hormone from working at the right times. Unfortunately, toxins and inflammation increase levels of reverse T3. Even if regular thyroid tests appear normal, high levels of reverse T3 mean your thyroid is not working properly!

Eat right for your thyroid. Limit soybeans, raw kale, and other raw cruciferous veggies, which might contain thyroid-blocking compounds called goitrogens. I know this sounds confusing. After all, I usually recommend plenty of cruciferous veggies. In this scenario, I am saying it's okay to eat them…just not raw! You should limit the kale juice and kale salad. One study in *The New England Journal of Medicine* looked at a woman who ate two pounds of raw bok choy a day and went into a hypothyroid coma!

I know that sounds extreme, but it could happen. I also recommend wild-caught, low-mercury fish, and seaweed for additional iodine – the mineral your thyroid hormones are made from. Since people eat less iodized salt, you might be iodine deficient. Over-exposure to fluoride, bromide and chlorine also create iodine deficiencies. Pumpkin seeds and oysters are excellent sources of zinc, and Brazil nuts provide selenium and iodine. Also, seaweed is a fantastic source of iodine and some varieties don't taste too bad.

Use quality supplements for thyroid health. A good multivitamin that contains the above nutrients, plus fish oil and Vitamin D, makes an excellent nutrient base. Some people may benefit from iodine supplements. Just be careful not to overdose and be sure to get your iodine levels measured regularly.

Replace the right thyroid hormones. Most doctors will only prescribe T4 (such as Synthroid), the inactive form of thyroid hormone your body must convert to its active form, T3. Most people do better on bioidentical hormones (like Armour, Westhroid or Nature Throid) or a combination of T4 and T3. A Functional Medicine doctor who understands how to optimize thyroid balance can customize a nutrient protocol.

Cortisol

Another source of weight-loss resistance is stress. Yes, you actually can think yourself fat or think yourself thin, and science proves it. Stressful thoughts activate metabolic pathways that cause weight gain and insulin resistance.

Cortisol is an adrenal hormone that helps you to run faster, see further, hear better, and pump fuel into your bloodstream for quick energy. It is the hormone that helps us survive in the face of true danger. It also shuts down digestion and slows your metabolism and increases Leptin resistance, making your body think that it is in a state of starvation (see beginning comments in this chapter).

All of this is perfectly normal in the short term, yet if left unchecked, prolonged stress and high levels of cortisol cause high blood sugar, increased belly fat, high blood pressure, high cholesterol, and muscle loss.

You can't eliminate stress completely, but you can reduce it with meditation, yoga, or deep relaxation, fun, tapping, dancing, socializing with friends, confiding in someone, praying or just listening to your favorite comedy show or music. These activities activate pathways that promote weight loss and health.

Sex Hormone Imbalances

Sex hormone imbalances, such as estrogen and testosterone, can also cause weight problems. Having too much estrogen causes weight gain whether you're a man or a woman. Do you know how ranchers fatten steer before they go to market? They implant them with estrogen pellets.

For both genders too much sugar, refined carbs, and alcohol spike estrogen. Keeping your gut healthy also cultivates healthy sex-hormone metabolism. Too little fiber or too many antibiotics damage the gut, triggering estrogen spikes because your body can't properly detoxify or excrete waste. Environmental toxins, like for example pesticides, are called xenoestrogens. This is because even at low doses, they act like estrogen in your body.

Symptoms of excess estrogen in women include breast tenderness, fluid retention, bad premenstrual syndrome, fibroids, and heavy menstrual bleeding.

In men, excess estrogen can cause loss of body hair (including chest, legs, and arms), a beer belly, and "man boobs." Low testosterone in men can also accelerate aging. Lack of exercise, alcohol, stress, environmental toxins or diseases like diabetes, and even pituitary problems can also lower testosterone.

Low testosterone causes men to lose muscle and gain fat, leading to sexual dysfunction, low sex drive, fatigue, mental fogginess, and bone loss that can lead to osteoporosis.

Interestingly, cholesterol produces testosterone and other sex hormones. Eating a low-fat diet and taking statin drugs that block cholesterol production can negatively impact your sex hormones.

If you suspect imbalances, you'll want to get tested.

These five strategies can help get you started:

1. **Eat a hormone-balancing diet.** The nutritional principles in *Eat Fat, Get Thin*, which is low in sugar, high in good fats, and high in fiber, can help balance hormones. Testosterone levels can increase 500 just by consuming healthy fats!
2. **Bulk up on fiber.** Fresh ground flaxseeds provide optimal fiber and lignans, which balance hormones. Even adding two tablespoons a day to a shake or a salad can help. You'll also want to eat fiber-rich organic fruits and veggies. But start slow on the fiber. If you are not used to it, it can plug you up.
3. **Foster daily elimination**. Constipation is bad for your hormones. Take magnesium citrate, vitamin C, probiotics, and flaxseeds daily to help maintain regularity. It's a foolproof combo for most people.
4. **Limit or remove alcohol**. Excess alcohol can compromise liver and kidney function, which inhibit detoxification and create hormonal imbalances, high triglycerides, and fatty liver.
5. **Get moving.** Exercise helps balance hormones, reducing estrogen and increasing testosterone, which helps you lose fat and build muscle.

Genetic Connections

Can our genes make us fat?

There are definitely some genes that can cause obesity. Though some of us may have the genes that predispose us to obesity and Type 2 diabetes, predisposition does not mean pre-destiny.

If you have a family history of obesity or Type 2 diabetes, or you are of Asian, East Indian, Native American, Pacific Islander or Middle Eastern heritage, you are much more likely to be carbohydrate intolerant. A little bit of sugar or starch will cause you to make way more insulin than others. This starts you on the vicious cycle of weight gain, hunger, and fatigue. The good news is that by eating well and exercising you can completely prevent obesity and Type 2 diabetes.

There are other genes that play a role in weight gain and weight loss as well.

The brain has genes that code receptors for dopamine, the pleasure producing neurotransmitter. Some of these genes cause the dopamine receptors to be less responsive to the pleasure signals provided by dopamine. Many drugs of abuse, including cocaine and heroin, trigger dopamine receptors.

The abundant abuse of drugs that are available freely and over the counter also triggers these dopamine receptors. These drugs are commonly known as “sugar” and “refined carbs”!

When your dopamine receptors need more stimulation to feel pleasure, it predisposes you to cravings and addiction. We know that sugar acts just like cocaine and drives food addiction and causes overeating. Dr. Hyman’s book, *The Blood Sugar Solution 10-Day Detox Diet*, provide a clear plan to break the sugar and carb addiction. But there are many ways to do this. Try starting your day with just protein and good fat for breakfast, salad for lunch and the starchy carbs for dinner with lots of veggies and see if this helps.

Other genetic factors also play a role. Just as different people have varying responses to carbs, they also have different responses to fats. This is new and emerging research, and more is being discovered every day. Some people do better with more Omega-3 fats, while some do better with saturated fats, and still others do better with more Omega-6 fats. Different people need different levels for balance. There can be a big difference in how your body responds to different fats and how they affect your blood sugar, cholesterol, and even gut bacteria.

The best consultant in the house is your very own body. Listen to that wise inner voice who gives you direct and immediate feedback about what works and what doesn't! So experiment, change it up, try different balances from one week to another or one month to another and see what works best for you. And your body changes as it gets older, so change with it.

Social Connections

Statistics show that we are 171 percent more likely to be overweight if our friends are overweight, but only 40 percent more likely to be overweight if our parents are overweight.

What does this tell us? Simply put: Our social connections are more important than our genetic connections in determining our health. The reason? Social connections influence our behavior. It's the power of peer pressure.

The way in which our environment and our social connections influence our health is what Dr Hyman calls *sociogenomics.*

Dr. Hyman, Pastor Rick Warren and Daniel Amen wrote *The Daniel Plan*, a faith-based wellness program that helped 15,000 people from Rick Warren's Saddleback Church to lose 250,000 pounds collectively, in 10 months, by doing it together. Rick says, "Everybody needs a buddy!"

Using the power of peer pressure for good can make it easier to do the right thing. So, set the example, eat well and let others follow. Be a food leader in your social circle! That is the way to institute change!

So, you can see it's important to surround yourself with healthy people if possible or join a community of healthy, like-minded people.

Those are my top tips for addressing a weight loss plateau. There is always something you can do. We can always dig a little deeper. And, if you feel like you're doing everything right and still not losing the desired weight, I highly encourage working with a Functional Medicine practitioner or good health coach.

Liver/Gall Bladder/Lymph Flow Health

You cannot deal with fat correctly if your bile is congested and toxic. When that happens, all your fat flow and absorption through your intestine is impaired and everything starts shutting down, including protein digestion and stomach acid production. Then your lymph circulation picks up unwanted toxic fat from your intestine and starts depositing that in your fat cells around your stomach and other locations, to protect the rest of your body. This is where eating good fats and liver/gall bladder flushes come in, clearing out old stagnant bile and fats, and getting your whole fat digestion and lymph system back on line (see my chapter on Detox). This is very important!!

Had enough? Whew…that was a lot of stuff. Just a couple more things…

Passive vs. Active Weight Loss: If you build your muscle mass up, you can be just sitting there and losing weight, because the more muscle, the more mitochondria to burn more calories. That is passive weight loss. Of course, it takes energy to build muscle, so you are getting two effects for the price of one effort! Yahoo!

Finally, brown fat is way more energy burning than white fat because what makes fat brown? You guessed it…mitochondria! You can increase your brown fat through cold therapy, that is, going from hot to cold quickly, like jumping out of a sauna into a cold shower, or turning your shower from hot to cold at the end of your shower to finish up. It is a good idea to start the cold water on your legs first and give yourself a few seconds to get used to it, then work up your body. You will love the feeling when you are done.

OK, I think that is about it. Hope you enjoyed the read and were not too overwhelmed by all the different piece parts to maintaining optimum weight. Just take it a step at a time and the new you will emerge from the cocoon you have been trying to shed…

LAST THOUGHT BREAK: MY ONLY POEM

When will God Return?

I look around to observe mankind

And see with clarity what divides us all

Surely god is waiting for us to realize

Before rejoining with hugs and kisses,

Finally, finally... love enthralls

For how can the Divine support one or the other

Without offending those precious souls excluded

For all exist in the blessed kingdom of life

No one better than the other

Only artificial barriers creating images secluded

If we only knew how we were supposed to live

All with creative powers

Effortlessly sharing energy, health, joy, and well wishes

The seeds would be planted, the garden would grow

Paradise returned; bliss through the hours

Then, then, my lovely spiritual brothers and sisters

Then, perhaps soon!, may we be untorn

Resume our daily conversations with god, mother earth and all that enrich us

Then will we be living the promise, the destiny of man fulfilled

No artificial barriers (race, culture, religion), Divine in all, the future reborn

CHAPTER 24

Financial Health

Money is a big part of our lives in this, our current reality. Money is a vehicle to transfer energy from one kind of energy expenditure (yours at your work place) to result in someone else's use of that energy in different ways (energy used by the company or service that receives your money). As a result, your use of energy at the workplace can in part be spent to cover your basic living needs at home. So, you take your creative energies, your emotional energies, your cellular energies and spend them at your work place, then the system converts those energies into a form that captures those energies and transfers them into other material or non-material results, much like our body does with ATP. Our cells take sugar and/or fat and through a process, convert those compounds into "money" (ATP) that can be transported throughout the body to be spent in both material and non-material (heat) forms.

This allows us to pursue our creative goals in life, doing what we love, rather than expending energy to take care of our basic needs like hunting or foraging for food or building shelter. Money is linked to our emotional wellbeing. It can lead to feelings of comfort and peace and security and success. It can be a currency of giving and friendship, or of frustration and failure. It can incite feelings of competition and pit people against people, destroy morals, fight wars, or advance technology used for good in our society or result in increased national security. We need to recognize the implications of money on our health.

By now, you know that there is no separation between our mental health and physical health and money can influence both. Beyond the emotional considerations, money can buy you all the organic healthy food and supplements you need to prevent disease. There are direct psycho/physical aspects of health to money as well.

If you have been "let go" or find yourself out of work, the trauma can have huge implications at many levels on your emotional and physical well-being. Our society emphasizes employment and work and pay and self-motivation, independence and initiative. No one is going to take care of you in this country if you cannot take care of yourself. That is a consequence of capitalism rather than socialism or communism.

Given that economic construction, it is you who must realize that it is up to you to find yourself a new job and market yourself and your talents to people who you may not know you. This is a skill. Some people come by it naturally, many do not.

If you are the type that is not self-motivated or have no clear ideas about what type of work would bring you joy, or have health issues that keep you from working, or are simply low energy or the lazy type, you will have an especially hard time in our society with potential implications on your health.

Networking is a big part of finding a job you love. It is much easier to secure a job that you love if you know how to build those relationships that lead to a position that brings your joy instead of drudgery. And it is important to your emotional health to do something you love.

My brother is a master in teaching people the skills they need to move in the direction of finding employment in something they love. I highly recommend his book. It is available on Amazon and is called, *The Power Networking Strategy: The Personal Approach to Landing a Good Job.*

Here is the link: https://www.amazon.com/Power-Networking-Strategy-Personal-Approach/dp/1944913130/ref=sr_1_1?ie=UTF8&qid=1542470207&sr=8-1&keywords=jay+arbetter

CHAPTER 25

Wrapping It All Up

Connecting the dots means putting the pieces together to help us overcome the destructive aspects of our environment which are detrimental to our health. We were born with the inherent drive and right to health. Once we understand what is holding us back from radiant health, we can begin working to fix it. All we have to do is ACT! That is no small order. That is where most people fail. They know what to do. They just don't do it, or try it, or experiment, or become their own doctor, or take responsibility for their own health.

I don't know about you, but I hate the fact that people are profiting off my ill health, controlling my food to gain maximum profit with minimum nutritional value. As Mark Twain said, "It is easier to fool people than convince them they are being fooled." On the other hand, there is a tidal wave coming of good, healthy food that you pay more for, perhaps at a local market or through the internet, that will nourish the body and mind. Hopefully, it will overcome and win out over the other side, eventually lowering prices of the healthier foods, so all economic groups can afford to stay healthy.

Once we fully understand the laws of life and the science behind how to best nourish the body and soul, then, those who act on that knowledge can truly lead long healthy lives, be creative and happy, until such time they move on to whatever comes next.

Let it be so....

ABOUT THE AUTHOR

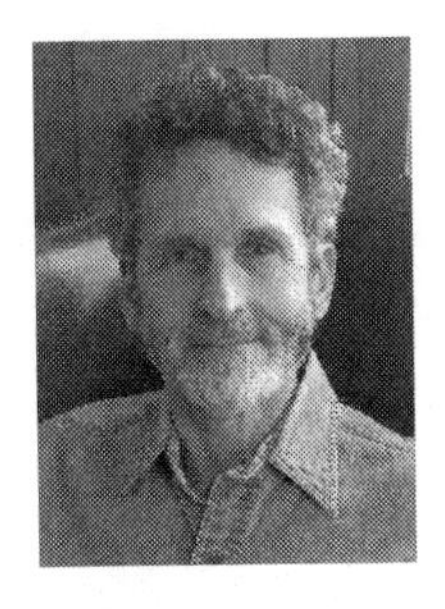

Dr. Bob Arbetter graduated from Texas A&M with a B.S. in Biology in 1976 and then served almost 26 years in various positions in the Air Force, retiring as a full colonel.

Having never lost his love for the biological sciences, he went on to get his PhD in Holistic Nutrition from the Natural Health University and then founded the Conscious Health Club so he could coach people to better health.

Bob is a board-certified Iridologist, helping people understand their body issues through analysis of the iris. He is married, has a step son and three wonderful grandchildren. He has helped many people regain their full health by uncovering the root cause of their various issues and then working with them in natural, drug-free protocols. His website and blog can be reached at Consciousheatlhclub.com.

38944582R00151

Made in the USA
San Bernardino, CA
15 June 2019